SYMPHONIES
— FOR THE —
SOUL

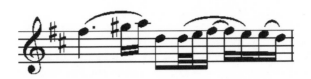

SYMPHONIES
— FOR THE —
SOUL

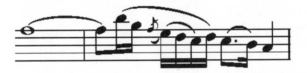

CLASSICAL
MUSIC
TO CURE ANY
AILMENT
— OLIVER CONDY —

FOREWORD BY JAMES NAUGHTIE

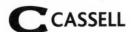

First published in Great Britain in 2021 by
Cassell, an imprint of
Octopus Publishing Group Ltd
Carmelite House
50 Victoria Embankment
London EC4Y 0DZ
www.octopusbooks.co.uk
www.octopusbooksusa.com

An Hachette UK Company
www.hachette.co.uk

Distributed in the US by
Hachette Book Group
1290 Avenue of the Americas
4th and 5th Floors
New York, NY 10104

Distributed in Canada by
Canadian Manda Group
664 Annette St.
Toronto, Ontario, Canada M6S 2C8

Instrument graphic: sashatigar/iStock

ISBN 978-1-78840-318-4

A CIP catalogue record for this book is
available from the British Library.

Printed and bound in the United Kingdom

10 9 8 7 6 5 4 3 2 1

Editorial Director: Joe Cottington
Creative Director: Jonathan Christie
Senior Editor: Faye Robson
Copyeditor: Diane Fortenberry
Senior Production Controller: Emily Noto

This FSC® label means that materials used for
the product have been responsibly sourced

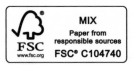

To Caroline, Alice and George

Contents

Foreword *by James Naughtie*

A characteristic of original ideas is that once they've been discovered, they often seem so obvious. Oliver Condy makes the point eloquently with this book. A guide to states of mind and to the music that might help – or *explain* – is an arresting thought, but also one that seems natural, and just right. Doesn't it reflect quite eloquently our own experiences?

Like everyone who will pick up this volume, I've had moments when I have needed a blast of something familiar. Or times when I've craved something new. But always with a purpose – to soothe or reassure, or perhaps to shake me up. Who doesn't have a particular recording of a Schubert song, or a Mozart piano concerto, or a Beethoven sonata, that they reach for in time of need? Who hasn't decided that a particular evening is the moment to put everything else aside and listen to a favourite opera, or the Bach cello suites, or a Broadway musical?

Although we enjoy music collectively – and who couldn't notice the exhilaration among musicians and in choirs when they began to perform together again after the terrible interruption of the Coronavirus pandemic – we are also aware that in times of anxiety or bewilderment, or in Condy's splendidly identified states of 'carelessness' (see page 31) or 'cabin fever' (page 29), we need music that speaks to us intimately, personally and, we like to think, with understanding.

I remember that the late Colin Davis, in his conductor's room at the London Symphony Orchestra, had a cartoon from the *New Yorker* on his wall that showed a barren moonscape, bleak and empty apart from a crushed-up Coke can and a few bits of discarded rubbish, and a bare horizon that promised nothing. The caption underneath read simply: 'Life Without Mozart'. Yet the truth that underpins this book is that the importance of music as a companion and a bulwark is not something understood only by those lucky enough to have a spectacular talent and a natural urge to perform. It's for everyone, even those who don't know it.

In his way, Oliver Condy was an educator when he edited *BBC Music Magazine* for so many years, because as well as highlighting the contours of the musical landscape around the world he was consciously introducing readers to music they might not know, or had forgotten. Composers who'd never popped up on their radar. A new pianist who might just turn the key in the lock and let them hear a familiar piece in an entirely new way. And that is the enthusiasm that runs through these pages – an urge to pass on the message.

Naturally, there will be arguments about some of these recommendations. *Really*? But he plays it so *fast*! She sang it so much better when she was *younger*! But that's half the fun, and it's testament to our connection with music that we love; it's part of the family, or a companion who must always be treasured. Every worthwhile journey involves moments of excitement, dread, disappointment and even melancholy. Happiness if you're lucky. Music is the expression of all these moods, and it is therefore a roadmap to a happy landing, and the next journey.

This book will have a place on my shelves where I can always reach it. For reassurance, solace, sheer excitement and fun. Most of us learn sooner or later that although music might not always provide an easy or an instant answer, it does tell us the truth.

Introduction *by Oliver Condy*

Music, oh, how faint, how weak,
Language fades before thy spell!
Why should Feeling ever speak,
When thou canst breathe her soul so well?
Friendship's balmy words may feign,
Love's are even more false than they;
Oh! 'tis only music's strain
Can sweetly soothe, and not betray.

From Thomas Moore, 'On Music', published in *Irish Melodies* (1807–34)

Music is a gift that nourishes the spirit in every possible way. That has been the view for hundreds of years, since the 6th-century BC philosopher, mathematician and pioneering musician Pythagoras was convinced that every planet in our universe resonated to its own 'music of the spheres'. Musical harmony, as he understood it, was even at the centre of our understanding of nature itself, all life on earth reflecting the character of the unheard celestial sounds. Hundreds of years later, Christianity adopted music as a sort of heavenly shortcut to God, while protest songs, particularly in the 20th and 21st centuries, have inspired us to stand up for our principles. The 19th-century Irish poet Thomas Moore, quoted above, neatly describes our enduring sense that music can access places other art forms cannot reach.

The 'ailments' we aim to remedy in these pages are all emotional. Music can heal a broken heart but has not yet been proven capable of healing a broken leg. While we suggest ways to treat your loneliness, grumpiness, feelings of regret and pangs of embarrassment, we cannot with any conscience help you with the common cold or a nasty rash. Nevertheless, music can nurse some serious emotional states and take you well along the route to healing. Some of our recommendations, including our cures for gluttony and exhaustion, are rooted in academic research; others have no genuine scientific basis, although we defy anyone with fully functioning ears not to be dragged into a state of joy by Mendelssohn's 'Italian' Symphony, one of music's sunniest and most optimistic creations. Where the ailments in question have veered towards the abstract – see the entries for rejection and betrayal – we have delved deep into the quirkier side of the composers and their music, offering anecdotes and life stories as doors to a sort of musical empathy.

As you explore the musical recommendations in this book and go in search of the right recording, you will soon notice that there are many to choose from. Often, pieces such as Beethoven's Fifth or Strauss's *Four Last Songs* will have been recorded hundreds of times, with even the same musicians having a second or third stab at them. These different recordings vary in speed, dynamics, instrumentation, recording quality and even, when a different performing edition has been used, in the notes themselves. We have pointed you towards the recordings we think are the very best, those that will provide you with what we think are the most faithful and pleasing interpretations. Our suggestions will save you hours of wasted listening. Perhaps the easiest way to listen to our recommendations is via a music streaming service such as Spotify, Apple Music or Tidal, or a specialist classical streaming service such as Primephonic or IDAGIO. But best of all is to build up your own collection of CDs or vinyl – physical manifestations of your emotional cures that can be with you whenever you need them, and a library on which you can continue to build.

And so we leave you in the company of some of the most beautiful and profound works ever composed, to help you find a musical path to contentment and emotional health. Happy listening.

Abandonment

Abandonment

George Frideric Handel's oratorio *Messiah* has become a companion to many over the centuries. Most choral singers can rattle off whole tracts by heart, while concert promoters will confirm its status as a guaranteed Christmas box-office hit. Like your best friend should be, *Messiah* is dependable and inclusive, rewarding to perform and uplifting to hear. Its arias, choruses and recitatives, telling the story of Christ's birth, passion and victory over death, are matchless in dramatic and musical quality – theatre and church have never been married so brilliantly.

Messiah's modern-day popularity is partly rooted in its early social role. London was at the centre of the burgeoning industrial revolution in 1742, when the oratorio was first performed. Global trade, huge wealth and innovation went hand in hand with massive population growth. But success also bred poverty for thousands of families who struggled to survive in London's heavily polluted, disease-ridden environment. For some children, the situation was especially bleak: many died or were simply left in the streets by parents who could not afford to care for them. Captain Thomas Coram, determined to do something, had received a royal charter in 1739 for his Foundling Hospital, a haven in London's Bloomsbury district where abandoned children could be nurtured and educated.

Central to Coram's success were the artist William Hogarth and the composer Handel, who in 1750 organized a benefit performance of his oratorio *Messiah* in the hospital chapel. The German-born Handel had by then been living in London for almost 40 years, writing works such as the opera *Giulio Cesare* and the *Music for the Royal Fireworks*, which in 1749 had attracted a crowd of over 12,000 to London's Green Park. Handel and Hogarth's sizeable contact books ensured that the performance of *Messiah* benefitting the Foundling Hospital was a sell-out, raising so much money that there were immediate calls for it to be an annual event. This came to pass, with Handel conducting every concert until his death in 1759. He left the priceless gift of a copy of *Messiah*'s manuscript to the hospital governors in his will.

Thus, even after his death, Handel did not abandon his beloved foundlings. And if you come to know *Messiah* – perhaps even to perform it – it will always be there for you.

RECOMMENDED LISTENING

Handel – *Messiah*

⊙ *Carolyn Sampson, Catherine Wyn-Rogers, Mark Padmore, Christopher Purves, The Sixteen/Harry Christophers (Coro)*

Acceptance (lack of)

The journey to acceptance is not always smooth, but submitting to an unchangeable situation brings wisdom, whether it be a frustrating everyday annoyance or, on a grander scale, fate itself. At least, that is the message in 'Saturn', one of the seven movements of Gustav Holst's *The Planets* suite. Holst was intensely interested in astrology, and rather than a physical description of our solar system, each of the suite's musical portraits is a sketch of the 'character' of a planet, as laid out in astrologer Alan Leo's 1912 book, *Art of Synthesis*. Mars, for instance, is the 'bringer of war – the wrath of God...that which is necessary to cause motion and activity', while Leo refers to Saturn as 'the subduer' and 'the bringer of old age'. 'None can neglect duty and escape the hard fate which Saturn imposes,' he continues – accept the path on which life has set you, he says, and you will gain a fuller understanding of yourself. 'Saturn' is the only movement in the suite that takes its listeners on a psychological and spiritual journey; it was reportedly Holst's favourite planet.

'Saturn' starts eerily, flutes rocking back and forth like the swinging pendulum of a clock, with a rhythm that infuses the whole movement. At its heart is a desolate procession shaped by an exquisitely crafted slow *crescendo* that grows from a weary, albeit very beautiful dirge to almost unbearable levels of despair, emphasized by indignant, insistent brass. Then panic, as a flurry of bells cuts through the procession, their confusion eventually surrendering to calm and serenity. The march fades into the distance, replaced by ripples and washes of sound, the orchestra giving way to a final, high *pianissimo* string chord that brings with it a mood of ultimate acceptance and serenity.

RECOMMENDED LISTENING

....

Holst – 'Saturn' from *The Planets*
⊙ *Royal Philharmonic Orchestra/Vernon Handley (Alto)*

....

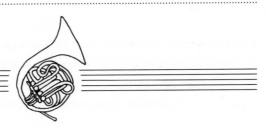

Adolescence

If we are being accurate, adolescence simply means one's teenage years, the time when girls and boys start to become young men and women. For some, however, adolescence has become synonymous with images of rebellious youths, reluctant to wash or enunciate beyond a grunt. For adolescents themselves, however, the truth is more confused – beneath the veneer lies someone in search of an identity and, ultimately, some sort of inner peace. An adolescent is on a journey. Some are further along the road than others but all are trying to prove their worth. Many of the great composers found themselves writing masterpieces just as puberty hit. Mozart is the most famous example of an adolescent come good, but he is certainly not the only one and, arguably, not even the finest. Take a look at a few genius adolescents – to restore your faith in the young and to give our spotty progeny something to aim for.

By the time he had turned 16, Camille Saint-Saëns had composed an oratorio, a collection of songs, a symphony and several cantatas. By 13, Dmitri Shostakovich was studying composition at the Petrograd Conservatory, exhibiting gifts 'on a level with Mozart', according to his teacher Alexander Glazunov. Just five years later, his talents had percolated down into the brilliant *Scherzo for Orchestra in F Sharp Minor* and sketches for his *Symphony No. 1* – works worthy of a great mature composer. And let us not forget Erich Korngold, who at the age of nine was proclaimed a genius by none other than Mahler and whose ballet *Der Schneemann* ('The Snowman') emerged when Korngold was just 13. It is worth hearing for its exquisite Straussian harmonies and complex orchestration.

Controversially, we shall skip over Mozart and turn to Felix Mendelssohn, whose *Octet*, incidental music to *A Midsummer Night's Dream*, string symphonies, operas, piano works (solo and concerto) and chamber music form surely the most staggering adolescent body of work ever written, all completed before his 18th birthday. If that is not enough to convince you of youthful promise, then there is no hope.

RECOMMENDED LISTENING

....

Mendelssohn – *Octet*

◉ *The Chamber Music Society of Lincoln Center (Delos)*

....

Adventure (lack of)

Whether pinned down by our jobs or submerged in family duties, many of us have missed the chance to embark on the adventure of our lifetimes. The irony, of course, is that when we were able to travel to exotic places, we did not have the means to do so. Help is at hand, however, thanks to several intrepid composers, including Béla Bartók, who in 1913 set off on a trip to North Africa.

Throughout his life, the Hungarian composer was curious about his country's musical heritage. As a young man he travelled the length and breadth of Hungary, noting down traditional folk songs and recording them on his phonograph. Bartók and his wife's trip to Algeria took things further: they ventured to the town of Biskra and its surrounding Saharan settlements before returning home armed with 65 songs on 118 phonograph cylinders. Their time there was not without incident: Bartók's request for local Tuareg women to sing to him was misinterpreted as a demand for prostitutes, while his wife complained that the local coffee had been made with dirty river water. Still, the centuries-old melodies he captured are mesmerizing – music of astonishing rhythmic and tonal complexity performed by singers and on wind instruments and percussion.

To satisfy your own wanderlust, you can travel alongside Bartók by listening to No. 42 of his *44 Duos for Two Violins*; despite its title, 'Arabian Dance', it is an almost direct transcription of one of these Tuareg melodies. Head next to the second movement, 'Allegro molto capriccioso', of his *String Quartet No. 2*, and you will hear the same hypnotic rhythms and wandering, chromatic melodies, complete with Eastern ornamentation. Throughout the movement, Bartók floats free of Western tonality and embraces his love of this traditional music.

Some 20 years later and 5,000 miles away, a young English composer called John Foulds was becoming disillusioned with European culture, travelling to India for a taste of its spiritual heritage and colourful, modal music. Western music, he realized, needed an infusion of outside influences to prevent it from becoming stale. He and his family headed to north India in 1935, giving recitals and training orchestras to survive, all the while collecting musical snippets from singers and instrumentalists in and around the Punjab. Many of the works written on his return have been lost, but you can hear Foulds's intense interest in Indian music in his spectacular orchestral work *Three Mantras*, an exhilarating piece replete with Indian modes and quarter-tone tuning that transports the listener.

RECOMMENDED LISTENING

Foulds – *Three Mantras*

⊙ *City of Birmingham Symphony Orchestra/Sakari Oramo (Warner Classics)*

sudoku

☆

7	2	5	6	1	3	9	4	8
6	9	3	7	4	8	2	5	1
1	8	4	9	5	2	3	6	7
8	5	6	1	9	4	7	2	3
3	1	7	2	6	5	8	9	4
2	4	9	3	8	7	5	1	6
5	3	1	4	7	9	6	8	2
4	7	8	5	2	6	1	3	9
9	6	2	8	3	1	4	7	5

Puzzle 15

Solution on 102

sudoku

★

8	6	9	4	1	5	7	3	2
1	4	3	8	7	2	9	5	6
7	5	2	3	6	9	1	8	4
3	2	1	6	5	4	8	9	7
5	8	4	9	3	7	2	6	1
6	9	7	1	2	8	3	4	5
9	7	8	2	4	6	5	1	3
4	3	5	7	8	1	6	2	9
2	1	6	5	9	3	4	7	8

Puzzle 14

Ageing

Old age can be approached either with a sense of excitement for the new dawn ahead, or with resignation, benign or otherwise. For musicians, however, it pays to look on the bright side. There is a simple reason why so many old classical musicians, particularly conductors, refuse to retire. It takes a long time to become a master of your craft, and most oldies still conducting orchestras will happily admit to only being half proficient from around the age of 70. In many cases, they are right. Italian maestro Claudio Abbado left the best until last, his final performances with the Lucerne Festival Orchestra producing some of the most radiant Mahler and Bruckner on record. And the late Nikolaus Harnoncourt, most famous earlier in his career for coruscating recordings of Bach, Beethoven and Schubert, let his hair down in the final years of his life with a blistering – and totally unexpected – recording of Gershwin's opera *Porgy and Bess*, made just months shy of his 80th birthday. Charles Mackerras's Mozart, Colin Davis's Nielsen, Roger Norrington's Beethoven – the list goes on.

It is not just conductors. There was a luminescence to Russian pianist Vladimir Horowitz's playing as he entered his final decade that you can see and hear in a solo recital from Vienna's Musikverein of Chopin, Liszt, Schubert and more – brilliantly performed at the age of 84. And at 82, the American pianist Leon Fleisher was made Instrumentalist of the Year by Britain's Royal Philharmonic Society.

Old age can often bring out the best in composers, too. Giuseppe Verdi wrote his operatic masterpiece *Falstaff* at the age of 79, having completed *Otello* just six years previously. Heinrich Schütz's astonishing *Schwanengesang* ('Swansong'), a collection of 13 choral motets, was completed when the composer was 86. At any time in history that would be impressive – in 1671 it was extraordinary.

But if any composer should convince you that old age is no barrier to success, it is the American composer Elliott Carter. Throughout his life, he had been a respected modernist, but in his final decade, Carter stripped away much of the complexity of his early music, finding a new clarity. The mercurial *Flute Concerto*, written at the age of 99, is a perfect example, as is the brief but mischievous *Dialogues II*, his final piece. He wrote it at 103.

RECOMMENDED LISTENING

Elliott Carter – *Dialogues II*

⊙ *Pierre-Laurent Aimard (piano), Birmingham Contemporary Music Group/ Oliver Knussen*

Anxiety

We all suffer from anxiety in one form or another. On a basic level, it can be a good thing – those butterflies in our stomach before a public event can help us achieve our best, whether singing, speaking, acting or performing. But at its worst, anxiety can be debilitating, manifesting itself in very real, physical ways. Most of the time, sufferers are aware of their anxiety's root cause, but many of us often live with the symptoms, unaware of what is behind it all. There are, however, ways to cope with anxiety, and one of them has been proven to be classical music.

A 2016 study in the *Deutsches Ärzteblatt International* journal compared the effects on blood pressure of Mozart's *Symphony No. 40*, a selection of waltzes by Johann Strauss II and various hits by ABBA. Before and after listening to the music, the 60 participants' serum cortisol concentrations, heart rate and blood pressure were measured. While the ABBA songs had little effect, the Mozart and Strauss resulted in falls in systolic blood pressure (referring to the maximum pressure your heart achieves while beating). Mozart also lowered heart rates, with Strauss coming a close second (ABBA, again, failed to score). Crucially for anxiety, Strauss had the greatest effect of all three on levels of serum cortisol.

There is no denying that the music mentioned above had positive effects, but there are surely better pieces to help bring feelings of anxiety under control. The opening of Mozart's *Symphony No. 40* – a nervous viola accompaniment underneath a tragic, minor-key melody – is the musical embodiment of anxiety; and Johann Strauss waltzes, while often elegant, do throw in some surprises from time to time. Neither seem especially conducive to lowering cortisol levels.

The *Deutsches Ärzteblatt International* study pointed to the following characteristics as being important for music to possess if it is to be of benefit for anxiety: a catchy melodic line, a pleasant key, skilful composition, few changes in volume or rhythm, harmonic sequences that are not 'rousing', and the absence of sung words. With those in mind, here are five listening suggestions to bring you calm.

Bach – 'Allegro', *Brandenburg Concerto No. 6*
Johann Sebastian Bach creates beautiful swaying rhythms in this gigue-inspired movement, scored for a rich combination of violas, violas da gamba, cellos and harpsichord.
⊙ *Concerto Italiano/Rinaldo Alessandrini (Naïve)*

Finzi – *Eclogue for Piano and Strings*
English composer Gerald Finzi's gentle, undulating piece for piano and orchestra was written in the late 1920s, and its pastoral character conjures up strong images of the English countryside.
⊙ *Martin Jones (piano), English String Orchestra/William Boughton (Nimbus)*

Chopin – *Nocturne No. 2*

The second of Frédéric Chopin's great *Nocturnes* takes the form of a slow waltz, with the composer's trademark vocal-like melodic lines soaring over the simple accompaniment.

⊙ *Nelson Goerner (piano) (Alpha)*

Tárrega – *Recuerdos de la Alhambra*

Francisco Tárrega's *tremolo* effect is a challenge for all guitarists to pull off, but it brings the shimmering heat of southern Spain and the 14th-century palace vividly to life.

⊙ *Alexandra Whittingham (guitar) (Delphian)*

Elgar – *Chanson de Matin*

Edward Elgar originally wrote this famous piece for violin and piano around 1889 and later orchestrated it. It is one of the composer's freshest, most appealing miniatures.

⊙ *English Chamber Orchestra/Julian Lloyd Webber (Naxos)*

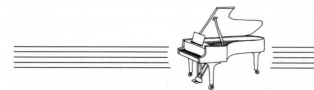

B

Bereavement

Choosing the right music to accompany the pain of bereavement is an almost impossible task, because extremes of emotion demand personal choices. Bach, Mozart, Beethoven, Schubert, Barber – all these composers have written music of great humanity and profound beauty, and each can help heal in its own way. There is, however, one work, blessed by a recording from 2020, that speaks with deep and direct empathy for anyone coping with the loss of a loved one.

When the poet Charles Silvestri lost his wife, Julie, to cancer in 2005, he and a close friend, the composer Eric Whitacre, embarked on an extraordinary choral work called *The Sacred Veil*, taking listeners on a heart-breaking and brutally honest journey from Julie's diagnosis through to illness, death and her family's bereavement. Silvestri's pain is felt all the more keenly because we witness, through his poetry and Whitacre's sublime music, the blossoming of the couple's love ('In a Dark and Distant Year'), the brief snatches of light and humour amid the darkness ('Delicious Times'), the prayers ('Dear Friends') and the final empty, hollow sadness ('You Rise, I Fall').

Silvestri's poems never flinch from the most personal, shocking details of his wife's disease, her symptoms, and the feelings of utter helplessness felt by her loved ones. Whitacre's music, scored for choir, cello and piano, skilfully and sensitively follows the contours of Silvestri's exquisitely told, heart-rending journey. *The Sacred Veil*'s final movement, 'Child of Wonder', features music of aching tenderness, setting a poem by Whitacre himself:

Child of wonder
Child of sky
Time to end your voyage
Time to die.

The oratorio ends on middle C, the note that represents Julie herself and the delicate veil between birth and death.

RECOMMENDED LISTENING

Whitacre – *The Sacred Veil*

⊙ *Los Angeles Master Chorale/Eric Whitacre (Signum)*

Betrayal

Forced into exile in 1849 for his (admittedly small) part in the Dresden Uprising, composer Richard Wagner was faced with the possibility that his music would never again be performed on German soil. But two people in particular stood up for him. One was Franz Liszt, who 'spoke with fire about the shame that Germany [had] abandoned his greatest modern composer'. The other was the popular French operatic composer Giacomo Meyerbeer who, even before Wagner's exile, had encouraged and promoted the young man and his music, introducing him to the director and principal conductor of the highly influential and important Paris Opéra. Wagner, in return, had written letters of gratitude to his 'deeply revered Lord and Master'. Back in 1838, Wagner had staged Meyerbeer's opera *Robert le*

Diable and later claimed it to be something of a model for his own works.

Beneath Wagner's obsequiousness, however, was a man full of racial hate. Wagner was anti-Semitic, and by the time he had returned from exile (with Liszt's financial help), his views on Jewish composers had been cemented, culminating in 1869 with the publication of his essay 'Das Judenthum in der Musik' ('Jewishness in Music'). One of the targets of his hate was Meyerbeer, whose successful opera *Le prophète* sparked in Wagner uncontrolled waves of jealousy. Meyerbeer's operas were, according to Wagner, nothing more than the corruption of high art by sordid commercial popularity. Wagner was biting the hand that had fed him, the hand that had promoted an early opera, *Rienzi, der Letzte der Tribunen* ('Rienzi, the Last of the Tribunes') and had helped get it staged in France and Germany. Hatred and betrayal would continue to be the deeply disturbing, ugly leitmotifs of Wagner's life.

It is perhaps fitting that the recommended music to hear in the face of wretched disloyalty should be the work that made Wagner incandescent: Meyerbeer's opera on the life of the Anabaptist John of Leiden, *Le prophète*, whose fizzing overture was rediscovered as recently as the 1990s.

RECOMMENDED LISTENING

Meyerbeer – 'Overture' from *Le prophète*

⊙ *Royal Philharmonic Orchestra/Henry Lewis (Sony Classical)*

Bewilderment

To newcomers, classical music can seem bewildering. Discerning the difference between a sonata and a suite, a symphony and a tone poem takes practice. Even the most seasoned of music lovers, however, are often left utterly bewildered by what is being performed for them on stage. Take Igor Stravinsky's *Rite of Spring*, whose far-out harmonies and jagged rhythms provoked a riot at its 1913 Paris premiere (see page 131). Or Arnold Schoenberg's atonal melodrama *Pierrot lunaire*, with its pioneering use of *sprechstimme*, or 'spoken singing', that scandalized New York at its premiere in 1923. According to one critic, the piece 'disrupted families, severed life-long friendships [and] incited critics to unbrotherly remarks about each other'. In 1927, otherwise progressive New Yorkers were again left scratching their heads when George Antheil's homage to modern methods of transport, *Ballet Mécanique*, was performed in Carnegie Hall. And no wonder: on stage were a siren, airplane propellers, a player piano, ten pianos, six xylophones and an assembly of other percussion instruments.

Today, it takes something truly odd to trouble concertgoers, but these five works from the 20th century are sure to puzzle anyone at first glance. As with much modern art, however, familiarity breeds understanding – with repeated listening, your bewilderment will be replaced by appreciation, if not passion.

Stockhausen – 'Helicopter String Quartet' from *Mittwoch aus Licht*

Karlheinz Stockhausen's *'Helikopter-Streichquartett'* forms a part of his opera *Mittwoch aus Licht* ('Wednesday from Light') and is scored for string quartet and four helicopters. Each musician rides in their own craft, naturally, and plays *tremolos* in such a way that their sounds blend with those of the rotor blades.

⊙ *Arditti Quartet plus helicopters (Montaigne)*

Young – *Piano Piece for Terry Riley #1*

La Monte Young's instructions for this piece include asking the performer to push a piano up against a wall – if the piano should go through the wall, then one is to keep pushing until the piano cannot be moved any further. Concert halls have not been particularly keen on this one.

⊙ *There are several very odd performances on YouTube*

Ferneyhough – *String Quartets*
Some will call the British composer Brian Ferneyhough's six string quartets among the most important pieces of the 20th century. But be prepared, as they are a sonic assault on the senses, and among the most complex quartets committed to paper. Persevere, however, and there are riches to be mined.
⊙ *Arditti Quartet (Aeon)*

Ligeti – *Poème Symphonique*
György Ligeti puts ten performers in charge of ten metronomes each. Wound to their limit and set to different speeds, the 100 metronomes are then left to tick away until, one by one, they wind down. The piece ends when the final metronome has stopped.
⊙ *Françoise Terrioux (metronomes) (Sony)*

Russolo – *Serenata*
Italian composer Luigi Russolo's *Serenata* sounds innocent enough, but the 1921 piece is a vehicle for the composer's *intonarumori* ('noises player'), a set of acoustic boxes that growl and roar in startling and not entirely pleasant ways.
⊙ *Fascinating early performances can be found online.*

Boredom

BBC Music Magazine ran a feature in 2011 revealing what its critics regarded as classical music's 'most boring pieces'. There was no doubt the list was controversial, containing pieces that many of us consider to be utterly engaging. Wagner's operatic reflection on love, *Tristan and Isolde*, was named and shamed for being 'the sound equivalent to water torture', while Brahms's *Requiem*, which many consider to be among the composer's most affecting and personal works, was dismissed as a 'soup of vapid consolation'. Also in the critics' sights were Purcell's innovative opera *Dido and Aeneas* ('it renders me still with ennui'), Mahler's mighty *Symphony No. 8* ('trickery without the magic') and even Puccini's most famous opera, *Madam Butterfly* ('we wait, and the waiting is long').

But what makes a piece of music boring? Its over-familiarity, perhaps? Mozart's *Eine kleine Nachtmusik* for string orchestra is a slice of sparkling wit and natural fluency, yet its over-performance in the 1980s and '90s has made it a tedious *persona non grata* ever since. For the same reason, Rachmaninov came to hate his own *Prelude in C Sharp Minor* – because it was played so often in the composer's presence, he grew irritated and bored with it. 'Many, many times I wish I had never written it,' he admitted. Or could it be that a piece simply might not chime with us – it is not boring; we simply don't get it.

Remember when you were young, and your parents insisted that boredom was a figment of your imagination? That with everything around you – books, toys, crafts, music, the great outdoors – only a fool would sit twiddling their fingers? To this author's mind, the operas of Monteverdi are among the less thrilling works to have sprung from a composer's pen. Sitting through all three a few years back was a test of endurance. But then that is what taste is all about. If you find one work boring, you can do one of two things: realize that you might be wrong and discover the beauty within that so many others have found; or move on to something else. It is not as if the classical repertoire is short of pieces to interest you.

RECOMMENDED LISTENING

Mahler – *Symphony No. 8*
⊙ *Soloists and choirs, San Francisco Symphony/Michael Tilson Thomas (SFS Media)*

C

Cabin Fever

Composing is a solitary, desk-bound activity, and many composers have found an escape in strapping on their boots and getting out into the open air. Mahler would often be seen, hiking-stick in hand, wandering through the Alpine foothills, while Brahms would hop over to Italy to amble along the banks of lakes Garda and Como, hoping for inspiration from the Italian air and wine. Holst was also a passionate rambler, and he and Ralph Vaughan Williams often went on 15-km (c.10-mile) strolls through the Herefordshire countryside. No wonder, then, that wide-open spaces and dramatic landscapes find their way into classical music. From the grassy Great Plains of North America to the rolling green hills of England, here are a few pieces to inspire you to revel in the great outdoors.

Vaughan Williams was passionate about English folk song, and thanks to his extensive research and detailed cataloguing, the 20th-century composer was largely responsible for its revival. Many of his orchestral works, such the *Norfolk Rhapsodies* and *Five Variants of Dives and Lazarus*, are shot through with snatches of folk song, beautiful melodies that evoke an English rural idyll. In the bittersweet *The Lark Ascending*, from 1914, a solo violin follows the upward trajectory of a lark, warbling and chirruping as it soars over the countryside at the height of a midsummer afternoon, hazy slow-moving orchestral textures holding it aloft like sonic thermals. But it is Vaughan Williams's *Symphony No. 5* that captures

C

the beating, brooding heart of Constable's England. A gentle, uplifting work, its rhapsodic slow movement is shot through with ravishing washes of colour and those timeless, haunting folk melodies.

Vaughan Williams was hugely influenced by Russian composer Alexander Borodin's exotic harmonies and atmospheric use of his own folk traditions. And so we head thousands of miles east to the Russia–Mongolia border, courtesy of Borodin's rich 1880 orchestral tableau, *In the Steppes of Central Asia*. Over its eight minutes, Borodin trains his telescope on a distant caravan winding its way slowly through the vastness of the Gobi Desert, accompanied by the metronomic plodding hooves of camels and horses. As if guiding our travellers on their way, a distant cor anglais (English horn) calls out a plaintive Eastern melody across the steppe.

Carrying on eastwards from Mongolia, we eventually arrive in the United States, where Aaron Copland's 1945 ballet, *Appalachian Spring*, paints an affectionate portrait of newlyweds setting up home in the Pennsylvania hills. In its opening minutes, strings and woodwind gradually unfurl, welcoming a new day with soft, open chords, a lone flute heralding the sun, glinting off the morning dew. Copland's genius lay in blending his vivid portrait of a busy Shaker community, complete with square dancers and country fiddlers, with music that gestures towards the wide-open prairies.

RECOMMENDED LISTENING

....

Vaughan Williams – *Symphony No. 5*
⊙ *BBC Symphony Orchestra/Andrew Davis (Warner Classics)*

....

Borodin – *In the Steppes of Central Asia*
⊙ *Orchestre de la Suisse Romande/Ernest Ansermet (Decca)*

....

Copland – *Appalachian Spring*
⊙ *BBC Philharmonic/John Wilson (Chandos)*

....

Carelessness

French composer Maurice Ravel was a musical master craftsman, whose every note has its intended place. Nothing is superfluous. Such precision earned him the sobriquet of 'the most perfect of Swiss watchmakers', and like Swiss watches, his music was not only forensically composed but is exquisitely beautiful as well. One work, however, stands out as a supreme example of the intricacy of Ravel's music. At first listen, the orchestral *Bolero* might strike you as a maddeningly repetitive work that quickly outstays its welcome. In fact, it is one of classical music's most original creations, constructed in the most minute detail and featuring a gradual, almost agonizing build-up of musical energy that is released in a shocking change of key in the work's final bars.

Bolero begins with a *pianissimo* side drum, its insistent rhythm repeated over and over again, driving the piece forward to its final collapse. The melismatic Spanish melody that floats and trips above is swapped between flute, clarinet, alto saxophone, muted brass, wailing trombone and a variety of startling instrumental blends, the side drum reinforced as the music works its carefully constructed way to an overwhelming climax. A successful performance will ignore any temptation to interpret the work, instead following Ravel's musical directions to the letter, steady tempo and instrumental control allowing the unbearable tension and madness to unfold even as the music reaches fever pitch, its carnival atmosphere disintegrating into cacophony before the final fall of the guillotine.

Ravel's meticulous attention to detail can be heard in his piano music, too, where nothing is left to chance – it is almost as if a perfect performance relies on nothing more than playing the correct notes and following to the letter the composer's dynamic and phrasing directions. Of course, there is a good deal more to it than that – the suite *Gaspard de la nuit*, for instance, is one of the

C

piano repertoire's most fiendish challenges, demanding a flawless technique and supreme tonal control. But take a look at a Ravel score such as the *Sonatine*, and you will discover a world of crafted beauty.

RECOMMENDED LISTENING

Ravel – *Bolero*
⊙ *Basque National Orchestra/Robert Trevino (Ondine)*

Ravel – *Gaspard de la nuit*
⊙ *Pierre-Laurent Aimard (Warner Classics)*

Cowardice

These days, politicians, environmental campaigners and fashion gurus grace the covers of glossy weeklies. Back in the summer of 1942, it was 'Fireman Shostakovich' on the cover of *Time* magazine: the composer stared defiantly into the distance, his fireman's helmet the symbol of a city's courage and resistance during the Siege of Leningrad. Between 1941 and 1944, over a million people died of hunger and cold as Nazi forces starved Leningrad of essential supplies. Tales of great heroism emerged during the siege, even if Dmitri Shostakovich's fireman duties – including protecting the conservatory from incendiary bomb damage – were little more than symbolic. The Russian composer, deemed too precious to expose to the front line, was evacuated months into the siege along with the Leningrad Philharmonic. By then, however, he had written most of his *Symphony No. 7*, a work whose music is almost as inspiring as the story of one of its first performances.

C

The 'Leningrad' Symphony is scored for a huge orchestra of over 100 players, but in 1942, as the siege took hold and the city was emerging from one of its coldest winters, its artistic scene lay devastated. Amid the cultural wastes was the disbanded Radiokom Orchestra, whose conductor, Karl Eliasberg, was given the task of reconvening his orchestra and performing the symphony to its dedicatees: the people of Leningrad. Eliasberg soon discovered that just 27 members of his orchestra were still alive – and only 12 were able to play. A combination of appeals, promises of extra rations and the sheer dogged determination of Eliasberg, who cycled around the city in search of qualified musicians, produced an orchestra of 80 emaciated, exhausted players. The Radiokom Orchestra's former drummer, Dzaudhat Aydarov, was discovered half-dead in a morgue and nursed back to life in time for the first rehearsal.

The performance in August 1942, broadcast across the city to both Russians and occupying German forces, was a symbol of determination and bravery – a show of an indomitable Russian spirit in the face of probable defeat. And this was no ordinary orchestral work they were performing. Even under normal circumstances, Shostakovich makes considerable technical and musical demands. The first movement's sustained *crescendo* builds over the course of over 12 dramatic minutes from a simple, almost trite military march to a bombastic, exhilarating display of ferocious might. The symphony's slow 'Adagio' movement is one of the composer's most bittersweet, alternating between staggeringly beautiful and hopelessly bleak. But it is the finale that wins out, a movement that travels from darkness to light over its 20 or so incredible minutes – a portrait of a city's courage in the face of unimaginable horror, both then and (under Stalin) to come.

RECOMMENDED LISTENING

Shostakovich – *Symphony No. 7 ('Leningrad')*
⊙ *Royal Liverpool Philharmonic Orchestra/Vasily Petrenko (Naxos)*

D

Deceit

Deception lies at the heart of Tomaso Albinoni's *Adagio in G Minor*, a piece for string orchestra and organ that has become best known for its use in film, most notably in the First World War epic *Gallipoli* (1981) and, more recently, the heart-breaking *Manchester by the Sea* (2016). In both instances, the *Adagio* works thanks to an artlessly simple scoring that pairs its melody with richly textured harmonies, replete with bittersweet suspensions. In places, much like Samuel Barber's 1938 *Adagio for Strings*, it is almost unbearably beautiful.

Albinoni's *Adagio*, however, is not by the 18th-century Venetian composer. It is, in fact, a forgery, written some seven years after Barber's *Adagio* by Italian musicologist and Albinoni biographer, Remo Giazotto. Unveiling the work in 1945, Giazotto claimed to have transcribed the piece from a fragment of a manuscript discovered in the archives of the Saxon State Library in Dresden. His story was all the more believable given that the library had been destroyed by fire during the Second World War and because it was known that a large amount of Albinoni's music had been lost then. For the music world, the *Adagio* was a powerful symbol of a precious treasure rescued from the ashes.

But as time went on, Giazotto's guilt ate away at him, and when the Dresden library denied ever having had the manuscript in its collection, he admitted to being the *Adagio*'s composer. Even the idea of it being based on a simple ground

D

bass from one of Albinoni's trio sonatas has since been discredited. Giazotto died in 1998 without explaining his reasons for the elaborate hoax, which are all the more unclear because it was the only music he ever wrote. Two things are certain, however. First, Giazotto copyrighted the *Adagio* and would have enjoyed considerable publishing, performing, recording and broadcasting royalties. His estate will still be dining out on it. Second, ironically, Giazotto has done wonders for Albinoni's reputation. His music is a far cry from the lush world of the *Adagio*, and beyond Giazotto's deception lies a composer of considerable skill in the mould of Corelli or Vivaldi, whose operas, sonatas, concertos and sinfonias might well have remained unexplored were it not for a deceitful academic.

Of course, we're not pretending that deceit is ultimately a good thing – reviving a neglected composer's reputation is surely not an excuse to hoodwink a generation. Listening to the *Adagio* at least prompts reflection on its far-reaching consequences.

RECOMMENDED LISTENING

Albinoni (Giazotto) – *Adagio in G Minor*
⊙ *Orchestre de Chambre Jean-François Paillard/Jean-François Paillard (Erato)*

Depression

Suggesting music to alleviate something so devastating, so crippling as depression could be seen as glib. But so many pieces of music have been written by composers in the grip of mental distress that hearing them can bring solace and a sense that we are not alone in our suffering. Indeed many great composers struggled with the condition throughout their lives.

D

The naturalized-English Baroque composer George Frideric Handel was prone to extreme highs and lows – hypomania and subsequent depressions. Periods of overwork would be followed by whole years of unproductiveness, made worse in later life by blindness caused by an inept eye surgeon. Perhaps even more deeply impacted was the 19th-century Austrian composer Anton Bruckner, whose family predisposition for depression culminated, for him, in feelings of extreme loneliness and a compulsive nervous condition that compelled him to count the leaves on trees, stars in the sky, blades of grass and windows in houses.

Elgar, Balakirev, Berlioz, Rossini, Tchaikovsky, Grieg, Debussy – depression claimed all of them in one way or another. But the Romantic German composer Robert Schumann's case is particularly acute. Schumann grew up in a family of intellectuals, some of whom had been touched by schizophrenia and depression. The composer himself was a heavy drinker in early adulthood, an affliction exacerbated by a diagnosis of syphilis (see also 'Despair'). He had already ruined his piano career by inventing a contraption designed to improve the independence of each of his fingers – it crippled him – but syphilis was at the root of his life of turmoil. Hallucinations and imagined sounds caused by the disease's effects on his brain resulted in near-constant depression and conspired to bring him to the brink of madness. Schumann tried to drown himself in the Rhine in 1854 but was rescued and thereafter confined to an asylum, where he died at the age of 46.

Throughout his tortured life, however, Schumann wrote exquisite piano and chamber music that only now and again offers glimpses of a man in extreme distress. Much of it is ebullient, virtuosic, heartfelt, generous music; but one collection of piano works, the *Gesänge der Frühe* ('Songs of Dawn'), written five months before his attempted suicide, embodies the spirit of a man whose music soars above his suffering. Described by his wife, Clara, as 'hard to understand' and 'so very strange', these admittedly startling pieces begin in almost unbearably beautiful religious solemnity with music that is simultaneously graceful and exuberant. The work's final chord, with its suspended note, is poignantly enigmatic. Everything about Schumann is here, his genius intact to the end.

RECOMMENDED LISTENING

Schumann – *Gesänge der Frühe*
⊙ *Piotr Anderszewski (piano) (Erato)*

Despair

It is not hard to find despair in classical music – the 'Adagio' from Beethoven's *Piano Sonata No. 29* ('*Hammerklavier*') underlines the pain of a man composing while almost completely deaf, while many of the slow movements from Shostakovich's symphonies are bleak, despondent reactions to Soviet social injustice. Few works, however, express feelings of personal hopelessness as acutely as Franz Schubert's *String Quartet No. 14* ('*Death and the Maiden*'), composed in 1824 and the finest of his late quartets. Just two years earlier, the 25-year-old Schubert had contracted syphilis and was very soon experiencing the pain and depression that accompanied the then incurable disease (see also 'Depression'). In 1823, Schubert poured his anguish out into a letter to his friend, the Austrian painter Leopold Kupelwieser: 'I feel I am the most unhappy, most wretched man in the world. Imagine a man whose health will never be sound again and who in despair only makes it worse, not better. Indeed, imagine a man whose most shining hopes have come to nothing, for whom the bliss of love and friendship offers nothing but acutest pain.'

D

Death and the Maiden, named after its second-movement variations on Schubert's 1817 song *Der Tod und das Mädchen*, is a musical mirror to the composer's worsening mental and physical health, a tragic masterpiece that brings the fear of mortality bubbling to the surface. It is easy to point to the opening cries of pain, or the manic dance of death in the final movement's *tarantella* as the most obvious portraits of Schubert's deep despair, but it is the variations themselves that carry the quartet's emotional weight – Schubert's realization that the circumstances of his earlier song setting had finally come to pass, expressed in music of complex emotions. 'Pass me by! Oh, pass me by!' says the young Maiden to Death, in Matthias Claudius's disarmingly simple poem. 'I am still young!' Death replies, with chilling calmness, 'Give me your hand, you beautiful and tender form! I am a friend, and come not to punish… Softly shall you sleep in my arms!'

Schubert's beautiful variations begin in hushed fragility, the haunting theme heard unadorned, like a funeral hymn, before violin and cello emerge, their urgent, pleading descants played out against an underlying thrumming, insistent rhythm. The cello's dramatic *crescendo* leads the movement to a ferocious mid-point climax before Schubert's anger subsides, the chorale returning once more to bring the movement to a resigned close.

Despair is one of the most isolating of emotions, but in the company of Schubert you can find a kindred spirit, someone to carry you along your journey towards hope and optimism.

RECOMMENDED LISTENING

Schubert – *String Quartet No. 14 ('Death and the Maiden')*
⊙ *Jerusalem Quartet (Harmonia Mundi)*

Despondency

> If you can meet with Triumph and Disaster
> And treat those two impostors just the same...

Rudyard Kipling's poem 'If—', written around 1895, is a list of life tools, including this two-line nugget of invaluable advice: do not get too bogged down by despondency or failure. The global pandemic of 2020–21 was tough and saw many lose hope in the face of repeated lockdowns, dashed promises of freedom and loss of livelihood. The music that can alleviate feelings of dejection and disappointment need not be irrepressibly happy, though – no one can be forced to 'cheer up'.

Here are some pieces that gradually bring the sun out from behind the clouds, and that can ease us gently into a better place.

Elgar – *Symphony No. 1*
Fast forward to the final two minutes or so and witness one of the wonders of British symphonic writing. Edward Elgar's grand, noble melody returns, surrounded by incredible bursts of cascading strings and woodwind before the final, grandiloquent climax.
⊙ *Staatskapelle Berlin/Daniel Barenboim (Decca)*

Fauré – *Nocturne No. 6*
Gabriel Fauré's piano masterpiece gives one of his finest melodies a rich, Romantic harmonic treatment. Written soon after the death of his parents, Fauré's music has a reassuring air, with a middle section that veers towards the ecstatic.
⊙ *Stephen Hough (piano) (Hyperion)*

D

Beethoven – *Violin Sonata No. 5 ('Spring')*

From the opening note, Ludwig von Beethoven's sonata oozes sunshine, fresh air and goodwill, but there are also moments of passion and spirit. The short, mischievous and rhythmically challenging third movement leads into a finale of rare, quirky delight.

⊙ *James Ehnes (violin), Andrew Armstrong (piano) (Onyx)*

....

Bryars – *Jesus' Blood Never Failed Me Yet*

Gavin Bryars's affecting work superimposes a beautiful instrumental score over a pre-recorded track of a homeless man singing an old gospel hymn. The combination of the repeated stanza and the growing intensity of its accompaniment makes for a haunting and uplifting listen.

⊙ *Ensemble conducted by Gavin Bryars (GB Records)*

....

Ravel – 'Adagio assai' from *Piano Concerto in G*

At the heart of Maurice Ravel's sparkling concerto sits one of the most gorgeous and poignant slow movements in all French music. After a long solo piano introduction, the orchestra eventually joins for what can only be described as six minutes of musical bliss.

⊙ *Jean-Efflam Bavouzet (piano), BBC Symphony Orchestra/Yan Pascal Tortelier (Chandos)*

....

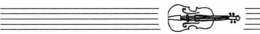

Devotion (lack of)

At sunrise on Christmas morning 1870, an ensemble made up of 13 members of the Zurich Tonhalle Orchestra gathered quietly on the winding wooden staircase of Richard Wagner's villa in Tribschen, overlooking Lake Lucerne, and began to play. The lilting music floated up to the second floor, where the composer's wife, Cosima, was dozing, waking her gently from her sleep. She later wrote in her diary:

> When I woke up, I heard a sound, it grew ever louder, I could no longer imagine myself in a dream, music was sounding, and what music! After it had died away, R came in to me with the five children and put into my hands the score of his 'symphonic birthday greeting'. I was in tears, but so, too, was the whole household...

Wagner wrote his *Tribschen Idyll*, known today as the *Siegfried Idyll*, as a loving 33rd birthday present for Cosima and as an expression of deep joy and gratitude for their son Siegfried, born a few months before their wedding in 1870. Wagner was entering a new period of inner peace, too, having put his first, disastrous marriage behind him. Understandably, the composer wrote in his own diary, 1870 was 'the happiest year of my life'.

The *Siegfried Idyll* was heard at various points throughout that day and was performed privately every year on Cosima's birthday until 1878, when Wagner allowed its publication to raise much-needed income. As an inspiring act of devotion, the *Siegfried Idyll* has few rivals, both for the quality of its intimate, delicate music — completely at odds with most of Wagner's output — and the circumstance of its first performance. But let us not forget the musicians who

D

rehearsed in secrecy, in their own show of artistic devotion. Conductor Hans Richter learned the trumpet specifically for the performance, reportedly rowing out into the middle of Lake Lucerne so that no one could hear him practise.

RECOMMENDED LISTENING

Wagner – *Siegfried Idyll*

⊙ *Bayreuth Festival Orchestra/Christian Thielemann (Deutsche Grammophon)*

Disappointment

To appreciate the best of life there have to be disappointments along the path, and nothing represents those low points quite as much as the inconsistency of the classical composer. Over the years, there been several high-profile discoveries of 'lost' works by great composers. Some have been found in libraries among the manuscripts of more minor composers, others have turned up in attics and dusty cupboards, while a few have emerged, blinking in the light, from the obscurity of private collections, having been kept away from the public gaze for years. It is always exciting to learn of a piece by Handel or Mozart resurfacing after so long, but the honest truth is that these pieces are often rather disappointing. A previously unknown *Allegro in D Major* by Mozart was uncovered early in 2018; it proved to be not much more than a fun frippery. And although a *Gloria* for soprano and orchestra by Handel, rediscovered in 2001, was initially said to have been so important as to 'rival *Messiah*', it was far from vintage. Soprano Emma Kirkby, who gave its first performance for two centuries, suggested that 'the piece has individuality and charm', with 'good bravura moments...'. Hardly a glowing endorsement.

It goes to show that even the great composers had off-days, their masterpieces tempered by plenty of duds. Here are five works that should have shown off the best of their composers, but which ended up as disappointing aberrations. Listening to these second-rate disappointments should only give you the confidence that fulfilment and success are just around the corner.

D

Beethoven – *Wellington's Victory*

Celebrating the Duke of Wellington's victory over Napoleon's brother Joseph at the Battle of Vitoria, this 15-minute piece should, by rights, have been as fine as Ludwig van Beethoven's *Symphony No. 3*, the 'Eroica' Symphony. Instead, it is a strange hotchpotch of popular songs, special effects and pointless bombast. Beethoven's response to criticism at the time is priceless: 'What I shit is better than anything you could ever think up.' It may have been a disappointing piece, but it made its composer a lot of money.

⊙ *Berlin Philharmonic Orchestra/Herbert von Karajan (Deutsche Grammophon)*

....

Wagner – *American Centennial March*

As did this rather drab piece by one of the great opera composers of the 19th century. In fact, the best thing about it, admitted Richard Wagner at the time, was the $5,000 he was paid to write it. Commissioned by the Philadelphia Orchestra in 1876 to mark the 100th anniversary of the signing of the Declaration of Independence, the 11-minute piece resembles something you might hear played at a graduation ceremony.

⊙ *Hong Kong Philharmonic Orchestra/Varujan Kojian (Naxos)*

....

Bach – *14 Verschiedene Canones*

What marks out the music of Johann Sebastian Bach is its incomparable marriage of sophisticated structure and aesthetic beauty, particularly in works such as *The Art of Fugue*, the *Goldberg Variations* and the *Musical Offering*. In these

14 imitative works (the title means 'various canons'), however, Bach bores for Germany, with clever but rather dull miniatures.

⊙ *Masaaki Suzuki (harpsichord) (BIS)*

Strauss – *Japanische Festmusik*

In 1939, Joseph Goebbels suggested Richard Strauss for the job of writing a piece to mark the 2600th anniversary of the Japanese Empire, for which Strauss was paid the modern equivalent of $75,000. *Japanische Festmusik* has some lovely moments, but the whole thing is very sub-Strauss: a collection of uninspired climaxes and wishy-washy textures that do not really hang together.

⊙ *Bavarian State Orchestra/Richard Strauss (Deutsche Grammophon)*

Tchaikovsky – *Fatum*

The symphonic poem *Fatum*'s first performance in 1869 was a moderate success, but its second outing prompted fellow composer Balakirev to write a harsh letter to Tchaikovsky, which he never sent. Probably a good thing, given that he referred to the work's 'cacophony' and suggested that it had been written in haste without much thought. Tchaikovsky destroyed the manuscript soon after, and it is very rarely performed today.

⊙ *Detroit Symphony Orchestra/Neeme Järvi (Chandos)*

Disdain

Wolfgang Amadeus Mozart was, on the whole, a tolerant man – even his love and respect for his father never wavered, despite an intense upbringing that included a relentless three-year musical tour throughout Western Europe.

By the time Mozart died in 1791, he was happily married, gainfully employed and at the height of his creative powers. He did, however, harbour an irrational dislike of the flute – which is a problem when you have been commissioned to write something for it.

In 1777, Mozart was asked to compose two concertos and a quartet for a wealthy flautist doctor. Exasperated by the idea of the task ahead, the composer wrote to his father: 'Of course, I could scribble all day long...[but] my mind gets easily dulled, as you know, when I'm supposed to write a lot for an instrument I can't stand.' Mozart may have had a point. The flute of this period – an unwieldy wooden instrument whose fiddly keyholes made it tricky to master, and a far cry from the user-friendly, multi-keyed metal instrument we know today – was seldom well played in the 18th century.

What eventually sprang from Mozart's pen the following year, however, were concertos the quality of which had never been heard before – or, arguably, since. Packed full of his most delicious melodies, Mozart's concertos challenge the flautist's technique and tone in the most delightful, playful manner, all wrapped up in fresh, artless music. The principal melody of his *Flute Concerto No. 1*'s 'Adagio' movement is among Mozart's most inspired, almost as if the process of writing it engendered a new love for the flute. (Unfortunately, it had not. In one of his more vulgar dispatches, Mozart's letter to his mother describes his plan of action regarding *No. 2*: 'The Concerto I'll write him in Paris, it's fitting, / For there I can dash it off while I'm shitting.')

RECOMMENDED LISTENING

Mozart – *Flute Concerto No. 1*
⊙ *Sharon Bezaly (flute), Ostrobothnian Chamber Orchestra/Juha Kangas (BIS)*

Embarrassment

In the mid-1920s, British composers Peter Warlock and E J Moeran moved together into an idyllic country cottage in the beautiful Kent village of Eynsford. That is where the idyll ends. In stark contrast to the beautiful pastoralism of their music, the pair wreaked havoc on their community. Tales of riotous drinking, sexual deviancy and drug-taking soon became the talk of the village, as Warlock and Moeran played host to the *crème de la crème* of badly behaved British composing talent, including Constant Lambert and William Walton. The good folk of Eynsford (a village with access to over 70 surrounding pubs) might have been a little more forgiving had the composers kept themselves to themselves. However, Warlock had the rather peculiar and, it has to be said, embarrassing habit of riding his motorbike through the main street of the village completely naked.

Rather less embarrassing was their music. Heavy drinking prevented Moeran from writing much in Eynsford, but his 1944 *Symphony in G Minor* is one of the glories of 20th-century pastoralism, making beautiful use of folk song from Ireland and Norfolk. On the other hand, Warlock seemed to find inspiration in drunken debauchery. To raise money for their Christmas booze, Warlock and a poet friend, Bruce Blunt, entered *The Daily Telegraph* newspaper's carol-writing competition. As Blunt recalled:

In December 1927, we were both extremely hard up, and in the hope of being able to get suitably drunk at Christmas, conceived the idea of collaborating on another carol which should be published in a daily paper. So, walking on a moonlit night between the Plough at Bishop's Sutton and the Anchor at Ropley [both pubs], I thought of the words of 'Bethlehem Down'. I sent them off to Philip [Warlock's real name was Philip Heseltine] in London, the carol was completed in a few days and published (words and music) in *The Daily Telegraph* on Christmas Eve. We had an immortal carouse on the proceeds...

Bethlehem Down is one of the most haunting and harmonically fascinating Christmas choral anthems ever written, but Blunt's account is shamelessly arrogant, and it would be nice to think that had he read it a few years later, he might have blushed a little. No one can deny, however, the poem's richness and resonant power, complemented perfectly by the aching tenderness of Warlock's lilting music.

There were more gems to come from among the empty bottles and cigarette ends. In Eynsford, Warlock also wrote the piece that would seal his place in music history. Just ten minutes long, the *Capriol Suite* is based on French Renaissance dance tunes and is a masterclass in subtle harmonization and string orchestration. Warlock brings a light, 20th-century touch to the dances while staying true to their 16th-century essence, as you can hear in the sublime, courtly fifth movement, 'Pieds-en-l'air', or the rollicking finale, 'Mattachins'. Clearly, great things can arise from outrageous behaviour.

RECOMMENDED LISTENING

Warlock – *Capriol Suite*
⊙ *English String Orchestra/William Boughton (Nimbus)*

Exhaustion

E

Go on – you can do it! Whether at the gym, simply trying to get through a day's work or bringing up a couple of squabbling children, exhaustion is never far behind. Music, however, has been proven to help rouse us: research points to the right kind of music reducing feelings of tiredness, increasing arousal levels, stimulating motor co-ordination and then, after all that, helping you relax. There is one condition, though – it is best if you are not working, exercising or juggling your life *too* hard, or your brain will not be able to concentrate on the music, and you will not feel the benefits.

An experiment carried out by professors from the University of Nottingham in 1999 hooked up a selection of participants to an exercise bike and a heart monitor. As each participant started to cycle, various edited extracts from Ludwig van Beethoven's *Symphony No. 7* were played to them through headphones. According to the research paper, the Beethoven work, featured in a 1976 performance by the Vienna Philharmonic under conductor Carlos Kleiber, was used for its 'exploration of the potentialities of rhythm throughout, thus making it suitable for such an experiment'. And indeed it is. Despite being written at a time of intense personal difficulties for the composer, Beethoven's Seventh Symphony is a work of high energy thanks to its dance-like rhythms, even in the grief-stricken second movement. Its final movement bounces with almost pure elation.

To the accompaniment of either the second movement, 'Allegretto' ('slow'), or the exposition of the final 'Allegro con brio' ('fast') movement, the participants cycled against a gradually increasing weight resistance. The results suggested that music was able to stave off exhaustion and increase stamina up to exertion at 70 per cent of a person's maximal heart rate reserve (MHRR), 'which is generally accepted to represent a borderline between moderate and high-intensity exercise'. The music, however, had to be of a suitably distracting character, with the fast extract outperforming the slower one.

So next time you feel the creep of exhaustion, pop on the final movement of Beethoven's *Symphony No. 7* and, with a bit of luck, you will carry on for a good while yet.

E

RECOMMENDED LISTENING

Beethoven – *Symphony No. 7*

⊙ *Vienna Philharmonic/Carlos Kleiber (Deutsche Grammophon)*

Failure (bouncing back from)

That one of classical music's greatest composers suffered a spectacular failure on the road to success is certainly a confidence booster. The 1897 premiere of Sergei Rachmaninov's *Symphony No. 1* was supposed to be the start of a promising career for the young Moscow Conservatory graduate. Four years previously, his one-act opera *Aleko* had been praised by no less than Tchaikovsky, rubber-stamping the composing career of a musician who could quite easily have made his fame and fortune as virtuoso pianist. Rachmaninov was riding high and spent most of 1895 on his ambitious new symphony.

Regarded today as one of Russian music's finest late-Romantic achievements, the First Symphony straddles the worlds of gypsy traditions and liturgical chant to mesmerizing effect – its final movement alone expresses a kaleidoscope of emotions, from its exhilarating opening to its tragic conclusion. But hindsight is a wonderful thing. In St Petersburg in 1897, an inebriated Alexander Glazunov, a better composer than conductor, was in the process of treading on Rachmaninov's dreams. The orchestra was under-rehearsed, and in concert the musicians could barely make out Glazunov's beat. It was an appalling performance. The composer sat on a flight of stairs outside the auditorium, covering his ears, waiting for the nightmare to stop. Critic and fellow composer César Cui publicly mauled the work, comparing it to the Seven Plagues of Egypt.

Rachmaninov was shattered and wrote practically nothing for three years. Money was tight, and he fell back on piano teaching to keep funds coming in. Finally, at a friend's suggestion, the 27-year-old composer visited the hypnotherapist and amateur cellist Nikolai Dahl, whose blend of hypnotism and gentle conversation seemed to break the deadlock; shortly thereafter, the *Piano Concerto No. 2*, which Rachmaninov had promised to London's Royal Philharmonic Society, flowed from his pen. The concerto is full of optimism, with achingly gorgeous themes and exquisite piano writing that never feels fussy or virtuosic for its own sake. It is a piece that oozes triumph over adversity – even apart from its history, its expressive beauty and defiant mood are inspirational. Happily, the Moscow premiere was a huge success, and Rachmaninov was back on track.

RECOMMENDED LISTENING

Rachmaninov – *Piano Concerto No. 2*

⊙ *Simon Trpčeski (piano), Royal Liverpool Philharmonic Orchestra/Vasily Petrenko (Avie)*

Faith (lack of)

Because of Christianity's place at the centre of European culture, Western music's first leap forward took place in church – specifically, Paris's Notre Dame Cathedral. It was there that two composers, the 12th-century Léonin and, 50 years or so later, Pérotin, used separate vocal lines in a bid to embellish the single melodies of Gregorian plainchant. This early polyphony would go on to be used spectacularly by the likes of Palestrina, Gibbons, Bach and thousands more. Ever since, composers have understood music's power to uplift us and its role in enhancing worship. Whatever your faith – even if you have none – these half-dozen works from across the centuries will inspire you with their incredible beauty and staggering craftsmanship.

Palestrina – *Missa Papae Marcelli*

Of the 100 or so Masses that Giovanni Pierluigi da Palestrina wrote, this one, composed around 1562 in honour of Pope Marcellus II, is his most famous. The music unfurls in an astonishingly natural way, in which nothing jars: the polyphonic writing is beautifully fluid, and each vocal line is in its rightful place. This is beauty on a heavenly plane.

⊙ *The Tallis Scholars/Peter Phillips (Gimmell)*

Tallis – *Spem in Alium*

Thomas Tallis's 40-part motet, dating from around 1570, is one of the most ambitious pieces in all choral music, scored for five eight-part choirs. Tallis creates moments of great intimacy, contrasting them with staggering, almost overwhelming climaxes of 40-part intensity.

⊙ *The Sixteen/Harry Christophers (Coro)*

Bach – *Mass in B Minor*

Arguably the greatest of all his works, Johann Sebastian Bach's setting of the Latin Mass was originally composed in 1749 as a job application. It contains music of both great solemnity and great joy – the 'Gloria' is utterly thrilling, the 'Sanctus' is majestic and regal, and the 'Crucifixus', with its staccato, hammering motif, is exquisite in its anguish.

⊙ *Collegium Vocale Gent/Philippe Herreweghe (Harmonia Mundi)*

Mozart – *Mass in C Minor*

Wolfgang Amadeus Mozart's most famous religious work is his *Requiem*, but the

Mass in C Minor for choir and orchestra is perhaps in a different league altogether. The opening 'Kyrie' and 'Qui Tollis' in the 'Gloria' are both infused with a tragic drama that even the *Requiem* cannot match, while the 'Sanctus' has a confident, Beethovenian grandeur. Inspiring from start to finish.

⊙ *Gabrieli Consort & Players/Paul McCreesh (Archiv)*

F

Parry – *Blest Pair of Sirens*
Hubert Parry's best-known Anglican anthem is *I Was Glad*, but this lesser-known, beautifully scored gem for orchestra and eight-part choir is a feast of glorious, soaring melodies and Victorian bombast. It was sung at the wedding of the Duke and Duchess of Cambridge in 2011.

⊙ *The King's Consort and Choir of The King's Consort/Robert King (Vivat)*

MacMillan – *Miserere*
A *bona fide* modern masterpiece, James MacMillan's work for unaccompanied voices from 2009 is his finest choral work to date, drawing on folk song, plainchant and Scottish rhythms. It contrasts its heart-on-sleeve beauty with moments of unsettling emotional rawness.

⊙ *ORA Singers/Suzi Digby (Harmonia Mundi)*

Fatalism

Ba-ba-ba-baaaaah... ba-ba-ba-baaaaah... 'Thus Fate knocks at the door,' Beethoven is reported to have said of the opening to his *Symphony No. 5*. Those eight hammering blows make up perhaps the most famous beginning to any piece of music in any genre, and represent what most of us imagine to be Ludwig van Beethoven the man – angry, frustrated, a composer who fought against the tide, a lonely revolutionary. There is every reason to believe that Beethoven regarded his 1804 symphony as a representation of mankind's struggle against the forces of fate. By the time he embarked on the work, he had begun to realize that his deafness would severely affect his life. And yet, if this incredible piece tells us anything about its composer, it is that he was determined to transform an impending disaster into a message of hope and optimism – victory over adversity.

The entire opening movement is dominated by the famous four-note motif that continually returns – transformed, overlapped, the mood both angry and despondent as each cry for help goes unanswered. A brief respite in the 'Andante' movement leads to the 'Scherzo', also coloured by the motif that gives it its unstoppable momentum. Towards the final bars of the 'Scherzo', however, Beethoven conjures one of the most miraculous passages in all orchestral music, beginning with soft taps of the 'fate' motif on the timpani, over which strings creep forwards, softly intoning snatches of themes we have heard elsewhere, gradually bringing the music out of darkness towards a distant glimmer of light.

Lesser composers may have instead used the silence between movements to effect a change of mood, but for Beethoven, this transition is where music meets theatre. His extraordinary transformation of the symphony from the key of C minor to C major signals the start of a final, triumphant victory that blasts forth in a mêlée of blazing brass, piercing piccolo, strident strings and thunderous timpani. Fate has been conquered by euphoria.

RECOMMENDED LISTENING

Beethoven – *Symphony No. 5*
⊙ *Vienna Philharmonic Orchestra/Carlos Kleiber (Deutsche Grammophon)*

Fear

Why is Johann Sebastian Bach's *Toccata and Fugue in D Minor* for organ so evocative of gothic horror? There is nothing particularly frightening or chilling about the piece itself. It is actually rather majestic – its opening descending octave scales, that dramatic spread diminished chord immediately after, and its stormy, whirlwind middle sections are fairly typical of the 18th-century pieces that aimed not to strike fear into their audiences but to explore every facet and pipe division of a north German organ. In fact, the work's fugue is nothing short of an intricate delight, beloved of both organists and listeners – not something to conjure up a scene from *The Phantom of the Opera*.

The piece's place in horror's Hall of Fame was initially guaranteed by its inclusion in the 1931 film *Dr Jekyll and Mr Hyde*, in which the toccata was orchestrated over the opening credits, and an extract from the fugue was tossed off by Dr Jekyll on his rather splendid house organ. From then on, a host of films used the piece to terrifying effect, including *20,000 Leagues under the Sea* (1954), in which the music was played by Captain Nemo (James Mason) on the organ built aboard the submarine *Nautilus*; the 1962 version of *The Phantom of the Opera*; the British horror film *Tales from the Crypt* (1972); and *Rollerball* (1975), in which the combination of pipe organ and dystopian science fiction created one of cinema's most menacing openings.

Ever since, Bach's *Toccata and Fugue* has been the musical shorthand for fear. At first, you should revel in a Pavlovian response to this wonderful piece – blast it through headphones and tremble. Soon, however, you'll begin to separate the beauty from beast, and instead savour colours and contrasts of one of the organ world's most alluring masterpieces.

RECOMMENDED LISTENING

RECOMMENDED LISTENING

Bach – *Toccata and Fugue in D Minor*
⊙ *Olivier Latry (organ) (La Dolce Volta)*

F

Forgetfulness

Listening to music can have remarkable effects on us. One of those is its uncanny ability to help us remember information. So thought Bulgarian psychiatrist Georgi Lozanov, one of the first to study music's effect on memory. His teaching method, known as 'Suggestopedia', uses background music not only to stimulate learning but also to help us shift whatever has been learned from short- to long-term memory.

There are three stages to the Lozanov method: relaxation, active learning and reflection. Relaxation puts the brain into a receptive state, primed for learning. Lozanov found slow Baroque music to be most effective for this stage. Then follows active learning, when more forthright music by Brahms, Mozart or Beethoven, for example, is played while you study and absorb information. According to Lozanov, bold, expressive pieces help the brain develop 'retrieval cues' that are linked to memory retention. Then comes reflection, a period of memory consolidation during which music can help once more with those all-important cues that will help you summon information during exams.

Listening to music while working takes practice, but if used in the right way, it may help you learn more efficiently and recall the facts and figures you need at the right time. Here are suggestions for each 'Suggestopedia' stage.

RELAXATION

Bach – 'Largo' from *Double Violin Concerto*

Johann Sebastian Bach's tender, descending melody weaves in and out of the solo instruments, accompanied by a gently pulsing orchestral accompaniment.

⊙ *Rachel Podger (violin/director), Bojan Čičić (violin II), Brecon Baroque (Channel Classics)*

Handel – 'Air' from *Water Music Suite No. 1*

George Frideric Handel's lilting 'Air', from music to accompany King George I on a trip up the Thames in 1717, is stately and soothing at the same time.

⊙ *Akademie für Alte Musik Berlin/Georg Kallweit (Harmonic Mundi)*

ACTIVE LEARNING

Mozart – Finale from *Symphony No. 41 ('Jupiter')*

Wolfgang Amadeus Mozart's final symphony is the culmination of his art – complex brilliance that wears its genius lightly. Listen to how the different voices interweave. Perfect for brain stimulation.

⊙ *Scottish Chamber Orchestra/Charles Mackerras (Linn)*

Brahms – 'Allegro' from *String Quartet No. 1*

A masterpiece that wears its heart on its sleeve, Johannes Brahms's First Quartet is contrapuntally thrilling, with something of interest in every bar.

⊙ *Belcea Quartet (Alpha)*

MEMORY CONSOLIDATION

Satie – *Gymnopédie No. 1*

Erik Satie effectively beat Debussy at his own Impressionist game with this

F

languid mini-masterwork, its exotic melody soaring over a gorgeous modal accompaniment.

⊙ *Noriko Ogawa (piano) (BIS)*

....

Rachmaninov – 'Vocalise'

Written for wordless soprano and piano, Sergei Rachmaninov's beautiful 1915 gem has been arranged for all manner of solo instruments and is both reflective and deeply passionate.

⊙ *Alisa Weilerstein (cello), Inon Barnatan (piano) (Decca)*

....

Forgiveness (difficulty with)

Two world wars and countless lesser conflicts and atrocities have meant that much of 20th-century culture has been defined either by anger and bitterness or by the search for reconciliation and collective forgiveness. Richard Strauss's searing and arguably greatest orchestral work, *Metamorphosen*, scored for 23 strings, was written in response to the bombing and resulting total destruction of historic Dresden in February 1945. Yet despite its overriding expressions of intense grief, anger and sorrow, Strauss's single-movement masterpiece edges towards resignation and relief.

There are similarly contrasting emotions in Benjamin Britten's *War Requiem*, composed for the consecration in 1962 of Coventry Cathedral, a symbol of hope for a city that, like Dresden, had been almost entirely razed by aerial bombing. The genius of Britten's oratorio was his interweaving of passages from the Requiem, the Latin Mass for the dead, with the bitter, disillusioned poems of Wilfred Owen. 'My subject is War, and the Pity of War,' Britten wrote on the cover page of the score, quoting Owen. 'The Poetry is in the pity... All a poet can do today is warn.' At its heart, however, is a message of peace and reconciliation. It was Britten's original intention at the premiere for the soloists to be from England, Germany and Russia: tenor Peter Pears, baritone Dietrich Fischer-Dieskau and soprano Galina Vishnevskaya. As it happened, the Soviets would not release Vishnevskaya, so British soprano Heather Harper took her place – although you can hear Britten's intended trio in the legendary Decca recording that was made soon after.

One of the most powerful expressions of forgiveness and redemption is the Seven Last Words spoken by Jesus on the cross. The seven phrases, extracted from all four Gospels, have been set to music by a number of composers, including Joseph Haydn (in 1787 for string quartet), Sofia Gubaidulina (in 1982 for cello, bayan/accordion and strings) and, perhaps most affectingly, James MacMillan, whose 1993 cantata for choir and strings, *Seven Last Words from the Cross*, is one of his most beautiful and moving works, born of a deep Catholic conviction. Its incredible opening movement is a musical summation of the pain, anguish, deep sorrow and forgiveness expressed in the simple phrase uttered by the crucified Christ: 'Father, forgive them, for they know not what they do.'

RECOMMENDED LISTENING

Strauss – *Metamorphosen*
◉ *Berlin Philharmonic/Herbert von Karajan (Deutsche Grammophon)*

Britten – *War Requiem*
◉ *Galina Vishnevskaya, Peter Pears, Dietrich Fischer-Dieskau, London Symphony Orchestra and Chorus, Highgate School Choir and The Bach Choir/Benjamin Britten (Decca)*

MacMillan – *Seven Last Words from the Cross*
⊙ *The Dmitri Ensemble/Graham Ross (Naxos)*

....

F Frustration

Pianist Glenn Gould called it 'just about the most astonishing piece in musical literature', while others have variously dismissed it as 'repellant'. Ever since its first performance in 1826, Ludwig van Beethoven's *Grosse Fuge* has divided opinion and caused more frustration among listeners, performers and musicologists than perhaps even the thorniest of atonal works. It is fiendish to play, hard to listen to, impossible to analyse. By the time Beethoven composed the work, originally the final movement of his *String Quartet No. 13*, he was profoundly deaf, somehow internally crafting each note. Beethoven's idea that such a piece – so long, so impenetrable – should follow the *Quartet*'s sublime fifth movement, 'Cavatina', seemed anathema to the audience at its premiere. He decided to retreat and write a fresh finale, publishing the *Grosse Fuge* as a separate work.

The 15-minute piece is ahead of its time, but the oft-repeated quote by Stravinsky that the *Grosse Fuge* is 'an absolutely contemporary piece of music that will be contemporary forever' cannot fully explain its power to disorientate. Its initial seconds are impossible to pin down: an opening octave leap quickly followed by a disjointed chromatic theme performed in unison. However strange, it is followed by a moment of calm as we enter familiar Beethoven territory – slow-moving, late Classical harmonies, hymnlike in their solemnity. Then a five-minute explosion of madness, as jerking leaps and counterpoint bombard at every turn, threatening to derail the music at any moment. It is exasperating to witness the music partially collapsing over and over again, each time struggling to regain control of itself. Finally, another moment of calm descends before Beethoven launches us skywards, disrupting the flow with barrages of trills. And then, as precipitously as a passing alpine storm, peace enters once again. The composer ends on a conciliatory note, teasing us with snatches of chaos before bringing us back to solid ground. Frustrations transformed into relief.

RECOMMENDED LISTENING

Beethoven – *Grosse Fuge*
⊙ *Belcea Quartet (Alpha)*

Fury

We all feel *furioso* from time to time. Sometimes the best way to alleviate rage is to wander into a forest clearing and scream. Not all of us, however, have forests to hand when we need them – nevertheless, listening to some of classical music's most furious pieces can have a similar purgative effect, particularly with the volume turned up.

For instance, has there ever been a more indignant, angry piece of music than the second movement 'Scherzo' from Dmitri Shostakovich's *Symphony No. 10*? The 20th-century Russian composer's frenzied portrait of Stalin has been called 'four minutes of rage' for its stabbing, violent rhythms. Or how about Polish composer Krzysztof Penderecki's *Threnody to the Victims of Hiroshima*, a nine-minute cry of unremitting anguish, the tone clusters in which take it to the very boundary between music and noise? Penderecki's demented music wails and shrieks, its deranged knocking effects and *pizzicato* adding to a dizzying, disorientating description of the horror of a nuclear blast.

Equally shocking is the expression of anger that emerged around 1935 from the pen of the otherwise placid Ralph Vaughan Williams, a composer famous for depictions of rural landscapes and for rescuing English folk song from extinction (see page 29). His *Symphony No. 4* is a blistering, violent and often bleak response to the then worrying situation in Europe, with Nazism well and truly on the prowl. Its opening minutes feature extraordinary waves of emotion that sweep over and engulf the listener.

Away from the anger caused by human injustice, composers have often tried to capture the awesome fury of nature. After witnessing the eruption of the Icelandic volcano Hekla, referred to in the Middle Ages as the 'gateway to hell', composer Jón Leifs was inspired to write one of the most terrifying pieces in all of classical music. Premiered in 1964, the nine-minute *Hekla* is scored for orchestra and a huge battery of percussion, including 'rocks with a musical quality', steel ship chains, anvils, sirens, church bells, shotguns and cannons. Never has there been a more intimidating piece, as Leifs's densely textured score explodes time and time again, musical fury taken to its absolute limits.

RECOMMENDED LISTENING

Penderecki – *Threnody to the Victims of Hiroshima*
⊙ *Polish National Radio Symphony Orchestra/Krzysztof Penderecki (Warner Classics)*

Vaughan Williams – *Symphony No. 4*
⊙ *London Symphony Orchestra/Antonio Pappano (LSO Live)*

Leifs – *Hekla*
⊙ *Iceland Schola Cantorum, Iceland Symphony Orchestra/En Shao (BIS)*

G

Gluttony

Next time you are in a fast-food restaurant, make a note of the music that is being piped in. Thanks to research carried out by Johns Hopkins University, the fast-food industry has discovered that loud, fast rock or pop music can encourage its clientele to buy more in its restaurants, and to eat more quickly. Expensive restaurants, on the other hand, realize that their customers prefer to savour their food, so they play music that feels unhurried and inobtrusive.

Researchers have seen a similar effect in supermarkets. In 1982, Ronald E Milliman, an American professor of marketing, published research into the way people bought their groceries, as well as the way they moved through the shop itself and the speed at which they did it. In contrast to the effect on fast food customers, Milliman found that shoppers in the American Midwest increased their spending when instrumental music of a slower tempo was played in a supermarket, as it encouraged them to move up and down the aisles more slowly and gave them time to remember everything they had come for; customers spent considerably less money and time in the store when faster music was played.

What are we to learn from this? If you are craving a Big Mac, then Estonian composer Arvo Pärt's beautiful, slow-moving piece for violin and piano, *Spiegel im Spiegel*, would be the perfect way to pace your enjoyment, give your stomach time to digest it and help you resist the temptation to super-size your fries.

For your weekly food shop, however, the fizzing overture to Georges Bizet's opera *Carmen*, followed by Franz Liszt's blistering *Transcendental Studies* for solo piano, will whisk you to the check-out in no time. In both instances, your powers of self-restraint – and your bank balance – will most definitely improve.

RECOMMENDED LISTENING

G

Bizet – 'Overture' from *Carmen*
⊙ *Scottish Chamber Orchestra/François Leleux (Linn)*

Gratitude (lack of)

Even the most successful composers have had to lean on the financial support of wealthy patrons, while having their confidence bolstered by the encouragement of close friends and loved ones. Some composers' dedications come from the heart, including Claude Debussy's modest inscription to his daughter, Claude-Emma, at the start of his piano suite *Children's Corner*: 'to my darling Chouchou, with tender excuses for all that will follow'. Frédéric Chopin, however, had social ambitions and enjoyed buttering up the aristocracy with dedications to dukes, countesses and various members of the nobility. And why not? What better way to express gratitude to someone than to link them forever to one of your masterpieces?

Perhaps the most heartfelt dedications are not from composer to friend, lover or offspring, but to a fellow composer. Music's progress has always relied on the baton-pass of knowledge and status, and acknowledgements of stylistic influence. Beethoven settled a musical debt to his teacher Haydn by dedicating to him his first three piano sonatas, as did Mozart, whose *String Quartets Nos 14–19* are named after Haydn. Maurice Ravel, still a student at the Paris Conservatory, paid homage in his *String Quartet* and piano work *Jeux d'eau* to 'my dear master Gabriel Fauré', the composer who set Ravel on his path and whose whispers of pre-Impressionist harmonic language almost single-handedly shaped French music well into the 20th century.

Ravel's 1903 *String Quartet* stands as proof of his appreciation, its music a golden bridge connecting the yearning, melodic Romanticism of late 19th-century French salon music with the thrusting, progressive harmonies and rhythms that would spring up in post-First World War Paris. Fauré was bewildered by the work, branding its final movement 'a failure'. Perhaps its dedication was as much a farewell to the past as it was an expression of Ravel's deepest gratitude to his once influential teacher.

RECOMMENDED LISTENING

Ravel – *String Quartet*
⊙ *Quatuor Ébène (Erato)*

Liszt – *Transcendental Studies*
⊙ *Kirill Gerstein (piano) (Myrios)*

Grief

Music can carry us through some of the most painful times in our lives, providing comfort and catharsis in equal measure. The music we choose to listen to when grieving is, of course, a personal matter, and much of it will be directly associated with memories of the departed – a Beethoven string quartet, a Brahms intermezzo, a Mozart symphony. Music can unite the past and the present, bringing with it a sense of time standing still and a space in which to reflect and heal. A favourite work can point to light at the end of the tunnel, too – a sense that things are going to be all right. These two contrasting masterpieces will resonate with anyone in the early stages of grief.

When Queen Mary II died from smallpox in 1694 at the age of just 32, England was plunged into collective mourning. Her funeral at Westminster Abbey was a lavish affair and featured Henry Purcell's extraordinary *Music for the Funeral of Queen Mary,* comprising a march, a *canzona* and three anthems. The music is so profoundly melancholy, so emotionally raw, that it is hard to believe that Purcell himself was not beset with grief. The introductory march, a cold, bleak lament scored in the tragic key of C minor for four trumpets and drum, is followed by radiant choral music, emotionally direct in its simplicity, from the major-key serenity of 'Thou Knowest, Lord' to the utter desolation of 'Hear My Prayer'. Its hushed, opening alto line begins a *crescendo* of almost unbearable tension, as Purcell builds up layer upon layer of counterpoint, falling motifs and harmonic dissonances, before culminating in a desolate open-fifth final chord.

Liberated from liturgical shackles, composers have often turned to the symphony to explore themes of life and death, but none more powerfully and personally than Gustav Mahler. The Austrian composer was haunted by death from a young age. The loss of several of his 13 siblings, his brother's suicide and, most devastating of all, the death of his daughter Maria at just four years of age meant that much of his life was shrouded in sorrow. Throughout his symphonic work, Mahler contemplates the nature of mortality, from the funeral march of his *Symphony No. 1* to a child's view of heaven in the divine final moments of his *Symphony No. 4*. However, the finale of *Symphony No. 9*, the composer's last completed symphony, contains music of searing intensity that hovers between acceptance and resignation, edging tentatively towards eternity in its dying minutes. On the score's final page, Mahler quotes a theme from the fourth song of his *Kindertotenlieder* ('Songs on the Death of Children') alongside the words 'the day is beautiful'. Even in times of great sorrow, he seems to say, life can still provide glimmers of hope.

RECOMMENDED LISTENING

Purcell – *Music for the Funeral of Queen Mary*

⊙ *Les Trompettes des Plaisirs, Lingua Franca & Vox Luminis/Lionel Meunier (Ricercar)*

Mahler – *Kindertotenlieder*

⊙ *Alice Coote (mezzo-soprano), Netherlands Philharmonic Orchestra/Marc Albrecht (Pentatone)*

Grumpiness

It is no surprise that so many composers have had a reputation for being a little grumpy. For a start, making a decent living from writing music has always been tough, and then you have musicians who will not – or cannot – play your music the way you want them to. There are the critics, too, whose opinions, to your mind, are utterly worthless, but who can make or break a career in just a few column inches. (Max Reger's notorious riposte to one writer is typically irritated: 'I am sitting in the smallest room of my house. I have your review before me. In a moment, it will be behind me.') If you are a genius, you probably will not suffer fools gladly, nor will you particularly care who you annoy. As Johannes Brahms famously said at the end of one social gathering: 'If I haven't offended someone here, I apologize...'

As a young man, Ludwig van Beethoven was frank to the point of hostility, with a proud streak that meant he was seemingly unwilling to conform or compromise. He had, however, good reason to be out of sorts. Increasingly deaf from a young age to the point where composing became almost impossible, he was also extremely clumsy. A friend and contemporary commented on his inability to pick anything up without dropping or breaking it. Beethoven's frustrations at his own bungling nature spilled over into the piano piece *Rondo in G Major ('Rage Over a Lost Penny')*. This grumpiness, however, was mitigated by an earthy humour. As Schumann wrote, the 'Rage' is 'the most amiable, harmless anger, similar to that felt when one cannot pull a shoe from off the foot...'

Finally, composers can be grumpy with each other. According to Beethoven, Rossini 'would have been a great composer if his teacher had spanked him enough on his backside'; Britten thought Puccini's operas were 'dreadful'; and Tchaikovsky considered Brahms to be a 'giftless bastard'. Still, given Brahms's own behaviour, he probably had it coming.

As we all know, grumpiness is a temporary state of mind. Turn to the beautiful, serene third movement from Brahms's *Symphony No. 3* and you will soon find yourself turning that frown upside down.

RECOMMENDED LISTENING

Brahms – *Symphony No. 3*
⊙ *Gewandhaus Orchestra/Riccardo Chailly (Decca)*

Guilt

As Picasso once said, 'Good artists copy, great artists steal.' And they don't apologize for it, either. 'Plunderphonics', a term coined in the 1980s, refers to pieces of music that 'borrow' from others. Some call these pieces 'homages', while others take a dimmer view and regard the idea of plunderphonics as outright theft. Composers borrow from each other (and from themselves) to varying degrees. Some might steal a chord here or a snippet of melody there; others might take a whole symphonic idea or a melody from someone else, and brazenly present it as their own. Remorse does not characterize those who practise plunderphonics.

There are forgivable instances in which composers, to save time, reuse and recycle – Handel and Bach, two prolific 18th-century composers, relied on reshaping some of their music for other purposes. Johann Sebastian Bach created two Lutheran Masses from church cantata movements, for instance, while George Frideric Handel forged new concertos and suites from the tunes of many of his own opera arias. Slightly less moral was the way Handel parodied the work of many of his contemporaries, including the likes of Scarlatti (both Domenico and Alessandro), Telemann, Stradella, Muffat and dozens more. One eminent musicologist has gone as far as to suggest that Handel was incapable of coming up with his own ideas.

There are, however, borrowings that are rather too close to plagiarism for comfort, many of them hidden away in film soundtracks. One of classical music's most notorious examples is the second movement of Gustav Mahler's *Symphony No. 1*, which bears more than a striking resemblance to the third movement of Hans Rott's *Symphony No. 1*, written over eight years earlier, in 1880. Listen to the rustic opening of Mahler's movement, and note how remarkably similar it is to Rott's, in terms of both scoring and thematic material. In fact, all four of Rott's movements contain musical ideas that occur in Mahler's symphony, which only redeems itself through its vastly superior musical craft. But does the end justify the means? Overwhelmingly, I say, yes – without Mahler's symphony, it's doubtful we would now be listening to Rott's. Mahler can walk away, guilt-free, with his head held high.

RECOMMENDED LISTENING

Rott – *Symphony No. 1*
⊙ *Gürzenich-Orchester Köln/Christopher Ward (Capriccio)*

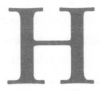

Hangover

The morning after is traditionally best greeted with a large Bloody Mary, a greasy fry-up, gallons of coffee and silence. It has, however, been proven that the right kind of music can help relieve the symptoms of a hangover. A 2011 study by Edinburgh University suggested that listening to certain types of music is better for mitigating the pain of a pounding headache and waves of nausea than any other activity, including sitting in silence. The theory, the study suggests, is that music not only provides a distraction from your discomfort, but that your emotional engagement with the music can change how your central nervous system receives those pain signals. The painkilling music, however, must express general contentment, be mostly bright in mood and certainly be in a major key.

Here are five pieces of delightful music to listen to as you grapple with your hangover and repent of your actions the previous night.

Mozart – 'Overture' to *The Marriage of Figaro*
Wolfgang Amadeus Mozart's 1786 comic opera begins with scampering strings that create a buzz of anticipation before trumpets and drums explode with music of pure and unbridled joy.
⊙ *Philharmonia Orchestra/David Parry (Chandos)*

Prokofiev – *Symphony No. 1 ('Classical')*
Fast-forward 130 years or so, and Sergei Prokofiev's First Symphony is an overtly sunny homage to Mozart and Haydn, with addictive melodies and beautiful, transparent orchestrations.
⊙ *Bergen Philharmonic Orchestra/Andrew Litton (BIS)*

Bach – 'Anima Mea Dominum' from *Magnificat*
Is there a more jubilant moment in music than the opening chorus from Johann Sebastian Bach's *Magnificat*? Drums, trumpets, strings and a chorus unite for a blast of Vivaldian exuberance.
⊙ *Monteverdi Choir, English Baroque Soloists/John Eliot Gardiner (SDG)*

Bernstein – 'I Feel Pretty' from *West Side Story*
Leonard Bernstein brilliantly captures Maria's confident optimism in this, one of the finest songs from his acclaimed musical. The orchestra trips along, gloriously carefree.
⊙ *Alexandra Silber (Maria), San Francisco Symphony Orchestra/Michael Tilson Thomas (SFS Media)*

Brahms – 'Allegretto grazioso' from *Piano Concerto No. 2*
In a masterstroke of breezy sophistication, Johannes Brahms matches piano writing of effortless grace with a rich, cosy orchestral accompaniment.
⊙ *Nelson Freire (piano), Gewandhaus Orchestra/Riccardo Chailly (Decca)*

Heartbreak (wallowing in)

Pyotr Ilyich Tchaikovsky's music feels like a compendium of lessons in love — whether expressing the first flushes of youthful passion in the sensuous main theme of the *Romeo and Juliet Fantasy-Overture*, or the hopeful outpourings of love in the Letter Scene of his opera *Eugene Onegin*. The Russian composer, however, wrote arguably his greatest work in the face of utter devastation. Towards the end of his life, Tchaikovsky, a repressed homosexual living in conservative 19th-century Russia, had lost all hope of ever finding love. Meanwhile, his patron, Nadezhda von Meck, who had supported him financially for 13 years on the condition that they never meet, had abruptly broken off their correspondence, ending a friendship that the composer valued deeply.

Heartbroken, Tchaikovsky set about writing his final symphonic masterpiece with surprising energy and enthusiasm, condensing his deepest sexual insecurities, forbidden loves and frustrated passions into music of astonishing power, vividness and unmitigated bleakness. *Symphony No. 6* was, Tchaikovsky wrote, 'the best, and, in particular, the most sincere of all my works', and was premiered just nine days before the composer's death from cholera, which was believed to have been self-inflicted after his illicit affair with an army officer was made public. Its opening movement, containing some of Tchaikovsky's most heart-rending music, swings between oases of calm and flashes of raging passion, a portrait of the composer's inner turmoil; the second movement, beautiful and delicate, is, in fact, a twisted, wrong-footed, damaged waltz, a misfit. An air of stoicism peeks above the parapets in the third movement march, a short-lived glimmer of hope before the 20-minute devastating finale that plunges the listener back into emotional depths.

For anyone going through the pain of lost love, the Pathétique Symphony is an empathetic travelling companion that will comfort and console.

RECOMMENDED LISTENING

Tchaikovsky – *Symphony No. 6 ('Pathétique')*
⊙ *MusicAeterna/Teodor Currentzis (Sony)*

Heartbreak (getting over)

Getting over the person that you thought might be the love of your life is not just about wallowing in self-pity. Yes, in the early days of a break-up, there is nothing like the music of Rachmaninov, Tchaikovsky, Chopin or Brahms to console you. As time moves on, though, the music you listen to needs to keep up with your changing emotions.

Here is music to take you on your journey as you pass from sadness and anger, to acceptance, to the final realization that you are free at last.

Purcell – 'Dido's Lament' from *Dido and Aeneas*
The ultimate accompaniment to loss. Henry Purcell proves himself a master of tragedy with this aria at the end of his 1688 opera. It adopts a chromatic bass line to devastating effect, while its sobbing melody is one of the most anguished in all of music.
⊙ *Lynne Dawson, Orchestra of the Age of Enlightenment/René Jacobs (Harmonia Mundi)*

Rachmaninov – *Variations on a Theme of Paganini (18th variation)*
The gorgeous, heart-melting melody that forms the emotional climax of Sergei

Rachmaninov's piano concerto is actually an inversion of Niccolò Paganini's original tune. Its major tonality gives it a sense of optimism and hope. One for the weeks following a break-up.

◉ *Nikolai Lugansky (piano), City of Birmingham Symphony Orchestra/Sakari Oramo (Warner Classics)*

Schubert – *Impromptu No. 3*

If you are not quite ready to move on, Franz Schubert's shimmering piano work is like a reassuring hand on your shoulder. Its yearning theme is tempered by a note of defiance that penetrates the calm. A magical glimpse of the happiness and inner peace to come.

◉ *Mitsuko Uchida (piano) (Philips)*

Mozart – 'Allegro' from *Clarinet Quintet*

Mozart's *Clarinet Quintet*, composed in 1789, has wonderful melodies, the best of which appears in the opening movement – 12 minutes of wistfulness combined with a sense of ebullient fun. This marks the point when you finally turn the emotional corner.

◉ *Martin Fröst (clarinet), Vertavo String Quartet (BIS)*

Mendelssohn – 'Allegro molto vivace' from *Violin Concerto in E Minor*

One of the happiest, most carefree pieces ever written, the scampering final movement of Felix Mendelssohn's *Violin Concerto* is entirely free of angst – perfect for sending you away with a confident spring in your step.

◉ *Maxim Vengerov (violin), Leipzig Gewandhaus Orchestra/Kurt Masur (Teldec)*

Hesitancy

Making the right decisions in life is all about pressing pause. It is all very well being decisive, but there is a fine line between a quick decision and impulsiveness. Cultivate a little more hesitancy in your life, and you may actually be happier with the paths you take. The same can be said about music. Sometimes the silences in a piece are more important than the sounds. Without the right space around it, music cannot reverberate, which in turn confuses its context and destroys its dramatic impact. Music needs to draw breath, to prepare itself for the moment to come. We all do. Here are five pieces in which the composer has used silence to extraordinary effect – a life lesson taught through music.

Haydn – *The Creation*
Never has silence been used to create such dramatic tension as at the start of Joseph Haydn's *The Creation*. Whispered by the choir, God's command, 'Let there be light', is followed by a short pause – enough for Haydn to draw breath for the light itself, which explodes in a joyful *fortissimo* chord of C major.

⊙ *Sandrine Piau, Miah Persson, Mark Padmore and more, Gabrieli Consort & Players, and Chetham's Chamber Choir/Paul McCreesh (Archiv)*

Rachmaninov – *Piano Concerto No. 3*
On a subtler note, Sergei Rachmaninov could easily have joined the second and third movements of his *Piano Concerto No. 3*, but instead he inserted the briefest of hiatuses. The silence gives way to a powerful downbeat that serves to kickstart the engine to a thrilling, virtuosic finale.

⊙ *Daniil Trifonov (piano), Philadelphia Orchestra/Yannick Nézet-Séguin (Deutsche Grammophon)*

Barber – *Adagio for Strings*
For seven minutes, Samuel Barber's work for string orchestra grows incrementally, building to a gigantic, sustained chord that breaks off, unresolved. And then silence. After what seems an eternity, a reply whispers an octave lower, and the tension is released.
⊙ *New York Philharmonic/Leonard Bernstein (Sony)*

Sibelius – *Tapiola*

H

In his last orchestral work, Jean Sibelius creates a profound sense of bleakness and isolation near the start, where a short, mournful orchestral phrase is answered by two whole bars of complete silence. The effect is utterly disorientating.
⊙ *Finnish Radio Symphony Orchestra/Hannu Lintu (Ondine)*

Beethoven – *Piano Sonata No. 8 ('Pathétique')*
In the coda to the first movement of one of his stormiest sonatas, Ludwig van Beethoven strips down the main theme, inserting dramatic and prolonged breaks that heighten the poignancy, each silence itself like an empty cry of despair.
⊙ *Stephen Kovacevich (piano) (Warner Classics)*

Hopelessness

There is surely no greater expression of hope than Ludwig van Beethoven's mighty Ninth Symphony. In the 200 years since its first performance, the composer's final orchestral masterpiece has morphed from a great German work to a musical monument of profound international meaning, performed at every conceivable celebration, from the opening of a major new music venue to the toppling of the Berlin Wall. It unites us all, crossing cultural borders and stirring quasi-religious fervour with music that thrills, delights, surprises and often overwhelms.

Emerging from almost nothing, as if painting the very moment of creation, the Ninth's first movement builds to a series of thundering climaxes before a second movement of pure electrical energy. Its expansive slow movement then lays the ground for the work's climax – a final-movement explosion of drama and jubilation in the composer's setting of Friedrich Schiller's poem 'An die Freude' or 'Ode to Joy', with vocal soloists and chorus at full tilt, united in their desire for universal brotherhood. That very idea must have sent shock waves at the work's 1824 premiere, not long after the French Revolution had failed and the monarchy had been restored. Sentiments such as 'All men become brothers' and 'Be embraced, ye millions' would have seemed impossible dreams.

This is precisely why we cling to Beethoven's extraordinary music at times when hope seems to lie within reach. In 1972, the Council of Europe chose the 'Ode to Joy' chorus as its anthem and, in 1985, European leaders adopted it as the official European anthem in three curious arrangements by Herbert von Karajan – for solo piano, wind orchestra and symphony orchestra – all of which succeed in removing the wind from Beethoven's sails.

Rather more musically on point, however, as the Berlin Wall was breached in

1989, ending almost 30 years of painful division, American conductor Leonard Bernstein led a performance of the Ninth, performed by an orchestra made up of the greatest players from around the world. Replacing 'Freude' with 'Freiheit' ('freedom'), Bernstein brought Beethoven's hopes to the surface, joy and liberty entwined as one.

RECOMMENDED LISTENING

Beethoven – *Symphony No. 9 ('Choral')*

⊙ *Members of various orchestras/Leonard Bernstein (Deutsche Grammophon)*

Humiliation

The trick to avoiding humiliation is to know your limits. Take, for instance, Louis Marchand, the great 18th-century French harpsichordist, composer and organist to the king. Quite a talent, you might think, but Marchand's downfall was his sense of superiority and lack of humility. Anecdotes of his temperamental behaviour abound, from plots to defame fellow organists to an extraordinary account of Marchand batting back Louis XIV's comments on his hands with an insult about the king's ears.

It is this lack of self-awareness and no little arrogance that led Marchand to agree in 1717 to an improvisation 'duel' in Dresden with none other than the formidable Johann Sebastian Bach. Competitions of this nature were common, with the winner judged to be the person to have given the most dazzling and inventive musical display. There is no doubt that Marchand had the potential to win – he was a master of the French style, which demanded a high level of spontaneity and free interpretation from its musicians. But Bach, despite being

German, was also a master of the French style, having studied as a child the French organ masters Raison, Couperin and De Grigny. He was also a master of the German style (naturally) and could compose Italian music better than any contemporary Italian.

On the day of the competition, Bach limbered up in front of the assembled crowd that included the king and his senior minister General von Flemming, whose palace was the ornate setting for the contest. Time ticked by, and Marchand did not appear. A messenger was dispatched to remind the Frenchman of the engagement, but to no avail. Marchand had escaped back to Paris by stagecoach without so much as an *au revoir*. The more charitable guests assumed that Marchand had gone to deal with an emergency, but the more knowledgeable among them suspected the truth. Marchand knew he was guaranteed to lose, and fled.

So, as a cure for humiliation, here's the perfect piece to warn us against overstepping our capabilities and embarking on challenges out of hubris. And what better piece than one of Bach's most perfect organ works – the *Fantasia and Fugue in G Minor* – improvised during his interview for an organist job in Hamburg. The remarkable thing about that is that this particular fugue is not only one of Bach's most beautiful creations, but also one of his most contrapuntally complex fugues. No wonder Marchand got cold feet.

RECOMMENDED LISTENING

....

Bach – *Fantasia and Fugue in G Minor*
⊙ *Peter Hurford (organ) (Decca)*

....

Humour (lack of)

It is not entirely clear why, but the French have always been good at mischief. Perhaps it is because ever since the French Revolution, they have been perennial experts at defying authority, their cabarets and clubs aimed at taking down the bourgeoisie. To outsiders, the French can seem a rude bunch – a misconception born of a mischievous sense of humour that is based on the put-down. In the first decades of the 20th century, while composers from other countries were concerned with such serious matters as how to adapt their music to the post-First World War order, the French shrugged and established Dada, an artistic movement mocking society and its absurd conventions.

If you are feeling a little humourless (or know someone who is) and feel the need for a spot of mischief to crack that smile, listen to these four French pieces for a little inspiration.

Satie – *Chapitres tournés en tous sens*
All mischievous roads lead to Erik Satie, king of musical Dada. This peculiar piano suite concerns a woman who talks too much, demands a hat of mahogany and rattles on so much that her husband keels over and dies from exhaustion.
⊙ *Noriko Ogawa (piano) (BIS)*

Poulenc – *Organ Concerto*
Francis Poulenc brilliantly subverts the organ's ecclesiastical role, opening with an irreverent parody of Bach and placing at its heart a superb evocation of a fairground organ. Explore more of Poulenc's work, and you will soon discover his marvellous sense of fun.
⊙ *Peter King (organ), BBC National Orchestra of Wales/François-Xavier Roth (Regent)*

Ibert – *Divertissement*

The ultimate mischievous orchestral work, guaranteed to bring you out in a massive grin. Concerning a hat that is eaten by the horse that is due to deliver a groom to his wedding, Jacques Ibert's music features a delightful mockery of Mendelssohn's 'Wedding March'.

⊙ *Orchestre de la Suisse Romande/Neeme Järvi (Chandos)*

Milhaud – *Le boeuf sur le toit*

Darius Milhaud's ballet ('*The Ox on the Roof*') is pure daftness from the start, its Brazilian influences and French silliness accompanying a scenario of a bar patronized by a little person, a bookmaker, a boxer, a woman dressed in men's clothing and a policeman decapitated by an overhead fan.

⊙ *Ulster Orchestra/Yan Pascal Tortelier (Chandos)*

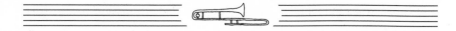

I

Ignorance

Ignorance can indeed be bliss – the more we know, the less we know, and with that comes the promise of a life of learning. If you do not yet possess much knowledge of classical music and how it works, then Benjamin Britten's *The Young Person's Guide to the Orchestra* is an ideal place to start.

To the uninitiated, classical music is shrouded in mystery. What is a sonata? A fugue? Who was Mozart? What makes up an orchestra? In 1944, the British government was asking similar questions and decided that music should be part of the national curriculum. The Crown Film Unit, part of the then Ministry of Information, was given the job of producing a series of educational films to complement government policy. One of those films was to be on the instruments of the orchestra, featuring music by Britten; he was regarded as ideal for the job, having already written the music for *Night Mail*, a documentary on the UK's postal trains.

The result was the 20-minute film *The Young Person's Guide to the Orchestra*, featuring the London Symphony Orchestra under conductor Malcolm Sargent performing one of Britten's most brilliantly inventive scores. Taking a theme by Purcell written in 1695, Britten concocts a series of dazzling variations on it, each showcasing different sections of the orchestra, from flutes and piccolos to double basses and percussion. The score ends in a blazing fugue that sees the instruments returning, in order, to play and reply to a mischievous invention by Britten, underpinned in the final minutes by Purcell's theme, performed resplendently by the brass section.

For those starting out on their classical music journey, the version with spoken narrative is recommended, although Eric Crozier's original script is hindered by its rather stilted manner. In which case, turn to Dame Edna Everage, who tweaks things here and there and, of course, adds her own inimitable style.

RECOMMENDED LISTENING

Britten – *The Young Person's Guide to the Orchestra*
⊙ *Dame Edna Everage (narrator), Melbourne Symphony Orchestra/John Lanchbery (Naxos)*

Impatience

Many of classical music's greatest works reveal themselves slowly. If you are the type that skips tracks if nothing happens within a few seconds, then know this: your impatience is denying you some fantastic musical experiences. All genres of music can stimulate the release of dopamine in the brain, the feel-good chemical that triggers sensations of joy and happiness, but pop music is rather too efficient. Like that chocolate bar that can give us an instant energy hit, it triggers multiple chemical boosts within just a few minutes. Too much of a good thing can ruin our sense of expectation and deny music's power to build dramatically over a longer period of time.

Here are five suggestions of mammoth classical masterpieces – the ones that will reward the hours of listening that they demand.

Bruckner – *Symphony No. 8*

One of the finest symphonies ever written, Anton Bruckner's masterpiece contains one of classical music's longest slow movements. But it is absolutely exquisite, shimmering, hovering expectantly, delivering tantalizing yet fleeting moments of pure heaven that eventually return for those willing to stay the course.

⊙ *Royal Concertgebouw Orchestra/Riccardo Chailly (Decca)*

Wagner – *Parsifal*

Pretty much every Richard Wagner opera runs into multiple hours, but it is the composer's Arthurian opera, the four-hour-plus *Parsifal*, that brings the most musical reward per minute. Over an hour into the action, Wagner places two of his most sublime orchestral passages: in the first 'Interlude' to Act I and then, after a further 90 minutes, in the 'Prelude' to Act III.

⊙ *Radio Symphony Orchestra Berlin/Marek Janowski (Pentatone)*

Mahler – *Symphony No. 3*

Gustav Mahler's six-movement hymn to nature is over an hour and a half long, moving from the harsh depths of winter to the composer's musings on what the flowers, animals, man, the angels and, finally, love can tell him. Its final movement is one of symphonic music's most glorious slow movements.

⊙ *Budapest Festival Orchestra/Iván Fischer (Channel Classics)*

Sibelius – *Symphony No. 5*

It is not so much the length of Jean Sibelius's most celebrated symphony that requires patience, but the beautifully crafted *crescendo* that stretches the entire length of the opening movement, starting with a gentle horn call from the mists and culminating in the final chord, a dazzling blaze of glory.

⊙ *Lahti Symphony Orchestra/Okko Kamu (BIS)*

Tchaikovsky – *Symphony No. 5*
You have to wait until the final two minutes of Pyotr Ilyich Tchaikovksy's
45-minute Fifth Symphony to hear the composer's utter wretchedness turn to
triumph. It is a hard-won battle, as the listener is taken through a despairing
first movement, a tragic slow movement, a melancholy waltz (does Tchaikovsky
write any other?) and, finally, the victorious prize.
⊙ *Russian National Orchestra/Mikhail Pletnev (Pentatone)*

I

Inadequacy

Feeling inadequate is emphatically not the same as being inadequate, and it is
generally a sign of low self-worth. That can result from a variety of damaging
experiences, whether they be overly critical parents or disparaging remarks
from your peers. The finest writers, painters, playwrights, poets and, of course,
composers all had to overcome misplaced criticism of their early works, after
which many picked themselves up, dusted themselves off and started again.
Some may well have given up, and we will never know who those were.

If you are feeling inadequate, try to filter out constructive criticism from
negativity, and do not lose faith in your considerable talents. After all, it is always
worth remembering that the record label Decca could well have ended one
young rock band's career with their damning rejection on the grounds that 'The
Beatles have no future in showbusiness.'

In that vein, here are four, now-much loved works that were initially marred
by criticisms so damaging that they could have single-handedly scuppered their
composers' future careers.

Howells – *Piano Concerto No. 2*

Herbert Howells was one of English music's great composing hopes, but at the 1925 premiere of Howells's Debussy-esque Second Piano Concerto, the critic Robert Lorenz stood up at the end and shouted 'Thank God that's over!' Howells retreated from the concert hall and spent most of his life from then on writing incredible music for the church, including anthems, liturgical settings and a breath-taking *a cappella Requiem*.

⊙ *Howard Shelley (piano), BBC Symphony Orchestra/Richard Hickox (Chandos)*

Tchaikovsky – *Piano Concerto No. 1*

Another piano concerto, but this time the criticism came from the pianist that Pyotr Ilyich Tchaikovsky had hoped would perform its premiere. Showing the score to Nikolai Rubinstein, Tchaikovsky waited for a reaction with bated breath. At the end of a long period of silence, Rubinstein declared the piece 'worthless and unplayable'. Nevertheless, it eventually came to be recognized as one of the great concertos in the piano repertoire.

⊙ *Denis Matsuev (piano), Mariinsky Orchestra/Valery Gergiev (Mariinsky)*

Elgar – *The Dream of Gerontius*

Unlike artists or writers, composers have to rely on musicians to put their music in its best light. Pity poor Edward Elgar, whose masterly oratorio from 1900 was almost derailed at the premiere by an ill-prepared choir and poor vocal soloists. 'I have allowed my heart to open once,' Elgar wrote to his publisher, Augustus Jaeger. 'It is now shut against every religious feeling & every soft, gentle impulse for ever.'

⊙ *Stuart Skelton, Sarah Connolly, David Soar, BBC Symphony Chorus and BBC Symphony Orchestra/Andrew Davis (Chandos)*

Bruckner – *Symphony No. 3*

It is a fair beast of a work at over an hour long, but the 1877 version of Anton Bruckner's Third Symphony was already doomed when its prospective conductor, Johann von Herbeck, died a month before the premiere. Bruckner stepped in, with disastrous results: by the end, most of the audience had left, and even some of the orchestral musicians had fled. Only 25 people were left listening to the end, including one Gustav Mahler.

⊙ *Gewandhaus Orchestra/Andris Nelsons (Deutsche Grammophon)*

I

Infatuation

The 1944 standard 'I Fall in Love Too Easily' could have been written for a number of composers: Johannes Brahms for his unrequited devotion to Robert Schumann's wife, Clara, with the result that much of his music oozes a quiet, simmering passion (see also page 104); or César Franck, whose *Piano Quintet* was written in an attempt to assuage his love for a music student of his, several decades younger. Contained within fellow Frenchman Hector Berlioz's major masterpiece, the *Symphonie fantastique*, is a vivid and often disturbing portrait of infatuation – perhaps the best that classical music has to offer.

It was a visit to see *Hamlet* in Paris one evening in 1827 that sparked the 23-year-old Berlioz's obsession. It was not Shakespeare who fired his imagination, however, as much as the actress playing Ophelia: Harriet Smithson. 'The impression made on my heart and mind by her extraordinary talent,' Berlioz later wrote, '. . .was equalled only by the havoc wrought in me by the poet she so nobly interpreted.' For days, Berlioz was in a love-struck trance, barely sleeping, wandering the streets of Paris. If his letters to Smithson were read, no replies were forthcoming. In a moment of hot-headed stupidity, Berlioz even arranged to live opposite her, watching her as she came and went.

Berlioz coped by putting all his energies into one of the most vibrant symphonic works ever written. The 'Episode in the Life of an Artist', as it was subtitled, charts the unrequited passion of a young musician, in mental agony under the harrowing influence of opium. Even when caught up in the swirl of a ball or escaping to the serenity of the countryside, the musician is unable to hide from his feelings of raging infatuation, highlighted for the listener by a short theme, or *idée fixe*, that pervades, even infects the symphony. Things end badly for the artist, of course, with murderous hallucinations and a witches' sabbath attended by his beloved, who dances orgiastically to the tune of the funereal 'Dies Irae'.

Berlioz and Smithson met in 1832 and married in 1833, but it did not last. What started as burning passion dissolved into bitter jealousy and resentment. Let that be a warning...

RECOMMENDED LISTENING

Berlioz – *Symphonie fantastique*
⊙ *London Symphony Orchestra/Colin Davis (LSO Live)*

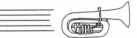

Insecurity

Today's world is more fractured and disconnected than ever. Social media has tricked us into thinking that the world is growing closer, but we have never felt lonelier. FOMO, 'Fear Of Missing Out', is a symptom of living our lives through our smartphones, which, in turn, takes us away from the here and now and damages our self-confidence.

Music, more than any other art form, is a great unifier. Singing or playing as part of a choir or instrumental ensemble brings huge benefits, including a feeling of belonging and a sense of collective achievement. Music, either performed or listened to, can galvanize nations, bring communities together and, in the absence of language barriers, cross continents. There is a reason why sports events and political protests place communal singing at their hearts – there is nothing quite like the feeling of belting out a football chant alongside 70,000 others. In the case of England's Liverpool Football Club, 'You'll Never Walk Alone' not only unites its fans in song, but links them in spirit, too.

If we are not singing or performing together, however, what music will make us feel part of something bigger? Are there pieces that can give us an increased feeling of safety and security? Much like scent, music is bound up with our memories. A song, symphony or choral work, perhaps a hymn you sang at school, can instantly whisk you back in time, bringing with it the emotions you felt at the time. It is what psychologists call a 'reminiscence bump' – a time machine for your brain – and it is why we often head for particular pieces of music to recreate those feelings. What is extraordinary is that music can work with dementia sufferers – in those whose short-term memories have been lost, music can reawaken their past lives in a seemingly miraculous way.

According to the eminent neuropsychologist Dr Catherine Loveday, many of our musical memories are bound up with our relationships – a song we listened to with a former lover, a piece of music played to us by a parent, perhaps something a grandmother used to sing in the kitchen. Music that takes us back to these times can have powerful effects. We even start to love the music that our parents listened to when they were young, because it reminds us of them.

This is where we depart from musical suggestions. Instead, reach out to that piece of music that makes you feel whole again, that wraps you in a warm blanket and lets you know that everything is all right.

Insomnia

As the story goes, the Russian ambassador to the court of August III at Dresden, Count Hermann Carl von Keyserling, suffered from terrible insomnia, and he asked Johann Sebastian Bach to write a musical cure – a set of variations on a simple bass line 'which should be of such a smooth and somewhat lively character that he might be a little cheered up by them in his sleepless nights'. The result was the *Goldberg Variations*, named after Johann Gottlieb Goldberg, a court harpsichordist whose job it was to play them from the Count's antechamber. It was a nice idea, but there was a flaw in the plan: Bach's music was just too interesting, for each of the *Goldbergs* is a sparkling, intricately crafted jewel. The music-loving ambassador would surely have found too much to enjoy and may well have spent whole nights in wide-eyed wonder.

For those of us who also struggle to fall asleep, there is a better, more modern solution. Yes, classical music offers a full range of soothing works, from long, soporific symphonic movements to hypnotism's musical equivalent, minimalism. And that is not to mention the lullaby, the traditional way to give parents a break. Max Richter's eight-hour, 31-movement sonic experiment

Sleep, however, is specifically designed to put you under and keep you there. For its premiere in the Reading Room of London's Wellcome Collection, audience members turned up at midnight, lay down on camp beds and drifted in and out of consciousness, lulled by the music's gently pulsing, soft-focus soundscapes. If any of them started snoring or talking in their sleep, they were not picked up by the BBC Radio 3 microphones. The live relay is, to this day, one of radio's longest single continuous music broadcasts.

How does Richter's music succeed when, say, Wagner's fails? While classical music does have its calming effects, there is always a loud section just around the corner, so unless you can guarantee falling asleep in less than 20 minutes, you risk being woken by a cymbal crash or brass fanfare. Richter, on the other hand, promises hours of unbroken bliss – and he has science on his side. After consulting with neuroscientist David Eagleman, Richter built the piece on low-frequency, repetitive sounds to reflect our brain's slow-wave state at night. Hours later, the music opens up, the high frequencies return and the listener wakes up, refreshed.

Although there is nothing stopping you from falling asleep to a Wagner opera, you will probably get a better night's rest if you follow the science.

RECOMMENDED LISTENING

Max Richter – *Sleep*

◉ *Max Richter (piano, organ, synthesizers, electronics), Grace Davidson (soprano), American Contemporary Music Ensemble (Deutsche Grammophon)*

Isolation

Musicians have always craved isolation, giving them the chance to practise in peace or work undisturbed on a new composition. Complete seclusion from the outside world used to be a luxury, and music's great masterpieces could never have been written except away from the incessant distractions of the day-to-day world.

Perhaps the most celebrated of today's musical hermits is the American John Luther Adams, composer of the hypnotic, sprawling, nature-inspired orchestral trilogy *Become Ocean, Become River* and *Become Desert*. Adams moved to the wilds of Alaska in 1978, living and working in a hut overlooking the mountains. It was a place, he later said, where 'the keynote is silence'.

Norwegian composer Edvard Grieg had a wooden composing hut built for him near a fjord in Troldhaugen, where he could work entirely undisturbed. Grieg was easily distracted – even the sight of a rowing boat would shatter his concentration. Gustav Mahler divided his periods of isolation between no fewer than three composing huts: two in Austria (Maiernigg and Steinbach) and one in modern-day Italy (Toblach). In Maiernigg, Mahler completed his *Symphonies Nos 4, 5, 6* and *7*, and much of *Symphony No. 8*.

The rather relaxed environment in which Grieg and Mahler composed is in stark contrast to Johann Sebastian Bach's more enforced isolation. In November 1717, Bach sketched out Book 1 of *The Well-Tempered Clavier* while imprisoned in Weimar, having allegedly broken the terms of his employment by expressing his urge to leave a court post and move to Cöthen. His sudden desire to write one of Western music's greatest keyboard works was, according to a local musician, one E L Gerber, the result of being 'beset by boredom and displeasure' and, of course, without an instrument.

In early 2020, national lockdowns bequeathed many of us enforced periods of solitude. For more than a year, auditoriums closed, travelling ground to a halt, and live music entered a period of hibernation. This was not the isolation we all wanted. If we glance back to those barren months, it is salutary to remember the glimmers of hope that shone in the darkness – artists who turned disaster into inspiration. There were remarkable broadcasts from artists at home, including the married duo of pianist Tom Poster and violinist Elena Urioste, who entertained thousands with their performances of music from practically every genre.

Post-classical composer Stephan Moccio's *Tales of Solace* represents a search for inner peace during this long period of isolation. A collection of 16 semi-improvised piano works, the album is performed on an atmospheric dampened upright piano. 'My piano's always been my confidante, my muse,' Moccio says, 'so I'm able to talk to her and have conversations.'

RECOMMENDED LISTENING

Moccio – *Tales of Solace*
⊙ *Stephan Moccio (piano) (Decca)*

J

Jealousy

Who can forget the moment, early in Peter Shaffer's 1984 film *Amadeus*, when Antonio Salieri, confined in his old age to an asylum, marvels with barely contained envy at the exquisite craftsmanship and seemingly divine melodic genius of Mozart's *Serenade No. 10 'Gran Partita'*?

> On the page it looked nothing. The beginning simple, almost comic. Just a pulse, bassoons and basset horns, like a rusty squeezebox. Then suddenly, high above it, an oboe, a single note, hanging there unwavering, until a clarinet took over and sweetened it into a phrase of such delight… It seemed to me that I was hearing the very voice of God.

Composers have always been jealous of one another, the emotion often manifested in snide and petty sideswipes. As Franz Liszt tried to impress a small, eminent gathering with his *Sonata in B Minor*, Johannes Brahms made a point of falling asleep, arguably in protest at Liszt's worldwide fame and notorious way with women (see page 143). Certainly, it is hard to believe that Brahms found Liszt's innovative, thrilling piano masterpiece boring. Sergei Prokofiev, on the other hand, once suggested to Igor Stravinsky's face that the opening to his ballet *The Firebird* contained 'no music'. The two were in constant battle over access to

Serge Diaghilev, impresario and founder of the Ballets Russes. What better way to attract positive publicity than to malign someone else's life's work?

It was not, however, a musical rivalry that provoked a 16th-century Italian composer to commit, out of pure jealousy, one of classical music's most heinous crimes. Carlo Gesualdo was born near Naples to an aristocratic family, but the young composer had no interest in politics, preferring to devote his life to music. When his older brother died unexpectedly in 1585, Gesualdo found himself heir to the family titles and married to his second cousin, Donna Maria d'Avalos. D'Avalos bore him a son but also indulged in affairs with several other men, among them the Duke of Andria. When Gesualdo caught wind of their relationship, he burst in on them together and murdered them in cold blood – along with, it is thought, his son – before putting their dead bodies on public display. It is a horrendous story made worse by the fact that Gesualdo's rank prevented him from being brought to justice, although he attempted to atone for his deeds by burning the forest surrounding his castle to the ground, and building a monastery and chapel.

Gesualdo's choral music is as tormented as the man himself. The sixth book of madrigals, written after his ghastly crime, is full of shocking chromatic harmonies, modulations and changes of mood that no other composer of the time would ever attempt. Listen to the grief-stricken 'More, lasso' for an insight into one of the most original composing voices of all time, and an anguished portrait of a man utterly destroyed by a fit of passion. May Gesualdo's music be a salutary warning against the powerful effects of extreme jealousy!

RECOMMENDED LISTENING
....

Gesualdo – *Madrigals*
⊙ *Les Arts Florissants/Paul Agnew (Harmonia Mundi)*
....

Joy (lack of)

My spirit sang all day, O my joy. Nothing my tongue could say, Only my joy!

Gerald Finzi, usually associated with a sense of reflective melancholy, wrote his exuberant choral setting of Robert Bridges's poem 'My Spirit Sang All Day' while courting his future wife, the sculptor Joyce (Joy) Black in the early 1930s. Finzi chose the poem for its constant repetition of the word 'joy' – for the composer, each 'joy' was a paean to his love. Not only was the piece created in the grip of pure happiness, but the music itself, written in the almost guileless key of G major, overflows with a sense of elation, right up to the final, ecstatic 'Thou art my joy!'

Even if music is not specifically about joy itself, nor contains as many mentions of it, it can still have the power to lift us up, to give us those feelings of utter delight that Finzi must have felt while composing his choral piece for his bride-to-be. Here are five other works to raise the spirits and, one hopes, keep them high.

Glinka – 'Overture' from *Ruslan and Lyudmila*
There are few orchestral works that are as utterly cheerful as Mikhail Glinka's overture. The music precedes the wedding feast of the opera's heroes, Ruslan and Lyudmila, and is a delight from start to finish.
⊙ *London Symphony Orchestra/Georg Solti (Decca)*

....

Holst – 'Jupiter, the Bringer of Jollity' from *The Planets*
Gustav Holst begins his ode to jollity with a sense of febrile anticipation – those bustling, almost muddled strings hovering above a forthright tune in the French

horns, before giving way to what can only be described as musical laughter. Then follows one of the greatest and most rapturous tunes in all of English music, a moment of pure bliss.

⊙ *Berlin Philharmonic/Simon Rattle (Warner Classics)*

Widor – 'Toccata' from *Organ Symphony No. 5*

No one, except organists, really knew of Charles-Marie Widor's spectacular organ toccata until 1960, when it was played at the London wedding of Princess Margaret and Lord Snowdon. Now it is one of the top choices for brides everywhere to sail down the aisle to – its rippling *arpeggios* and thundering bass are a perfect accompaniment to a blissful event.

⊙ *Joseph Nolan (organ) (Signum)*

Litolff – 'Scherzo' from *Concerto Symphonique No. 4*

At first listen, Henry Litolff's 'Scherzo' seems to be cut from the same cloth as the 'Allegro scherzando' from Camille Saint-Saëns's *Piano Concerto No. 2*, but this slice of virtuosic joy was written some 17 years earlier. It is the only piece by Litolff that remains in the repertoire today, but it is a cheery cracker.

⊙ *Peter Donohoe (piano), Bournemouth Symphony Orchestra/Andrew Litton (Hyperion)*

Bach – 'Prelude and Fugue in D Minor' from Book I of *The Well-Tempered Clavier*

One minute of pure delight, as a simple bass of bouncing quavers (eighth notes) forms the foundation underneath a babbling brook of semi-quavers (sixteenth notes). It is irrepressible fun, and it beautifully complements its fugue – an inventive, French overture-inspired piece that wears its stateliness lightly.

⊙ *András Schiff (piano) (ECM)*

K

Killjoy (being a)

You have accepted an invitation to one of the most hotly anticipated parties in living memory. Then the day arrives, and you would rather put your feet up in front of a new television series. What you need is a party animal to get you in the mood, and you could certainly do a lot worse than a composer. Many of us will have wined and dined before, during and after an opera or concert. And who has not listened to their favourite piece of music with the added accompaniment of a fizzing beer top or a popping cork? Leave aside real life for a moment, however, and delve into the world of the fictional party – the one that really zings and where everyone, yourself included, is great company. These are the parties that stay in the memory and, more importantly, get you out the door and into the party spirit.

You could start with, say, Giuseppe Verdi's *La traviata*, which opens with a grand *soirée* at the house of courtesan Violetta Valéry. 'Libiamo ne' lieti calici' ('Let's drink from merry glasses') is one of opera's most effervescent arias, but it is probably best to pause the music after its final bar, before Violetta starts to show symptoms of the consumption that eventually finishes her off. Violetta's is not the only operatic party to end badly. Benjamin Britten's Albert Herring, in the opera of the same name, finds himself in trouble thanks to a spiked lemonade drink, while in Leoš Janáček's *Jenůfa*, Steva and his fiancée indulge in some vigorous dancing, only for their fun to be spoiled by an overprotective mother-in-law.

Let us steer clear of opera and head to the beautiful, remote landscapes of Orkney, and a short dose of unadulterated orchestral delight. Not even Verdi does booze-fuelled celebration as well as Peter Maxwell Davies. Premiered in 1985, *An Orkney Wedding, with Sunrise* is a mere 13 minutes in length but covers the arc of a wedding celebration, from a stately procession at sunrise to drunken dancing courtesy of an Orcadian fiddler who can barely keep up. Guests, unsteady on their feet, head once more to the bar before the sun rises over the islands, bagpipes finally bringing the revellers to their senses. Who could resist a party like that?

K

RECOMMENDED LISTENING

Maxwell Davies – *An Orkney Wedding, with Sunrise*
◉ *Scottish Chamber Orchestra/Ben Gernon (Linn)*

L

Laziness

Are you lazy or are you, in truth, a perfectionist? It is very important to find your own pace of working – if school taught us anything, it is that we should not admire anyone who completes their work with suspicious speed. Of course, there are those utterly irritating people who can combine excellence and efficiency, but there are more of us who toil long hours to produce our own small but perfectly formed pieces of work.

This is why we should take heart from the music of Anatoly Lyadov, a Russian composer whom compatriot Nicolai Rimsky-Korsakov once called 'incredibly lazy'. He did have a point – Lyadov's inability to complete *The Firebird* for the Ballets Russes inadvertently gave Igor Stravinsky his big break. But that is only part of the story. Lyadov's reluctance to put his nose to the grindstone seems to have stemmed partly from witnessing his own father, Konstantin, work himself into an early grave as conductor of St Petersburg's Imperial Opera Company. But he was also easily distracted, preferring the company of his closest friend to the St Petersburg Conservatory classes of Rimsky-Korsakov – who summarily had them both booted from their course for missing too many lessons.

While he was playing truant, Lyadov was actually hard at work composing piano music of sparkling brilliance – Chopin-esque miniatures that display impressive craftsmanship, including a *Prelude in B Flat Minor* and a collection of short piano pieces, *Biryulki*. Years later, he would go on to write his greatest piano work, the *Ballade (In Olden Days)*, which sits alongside the best of Brahms's solo piano works.

Lyadov's failure to write his planned opera may have been down to sheer lack of motivation, but the truth is, we simply do not know. All that survives of the sketches to *Zoryushka*, a magical tale of a princess, her suitors and wood spirits, are two orchestral tone poems: *Kikimora* and *The Enchanted Lake*. Despite their briefness, both are wonderfully orchestrated, containing the very best of Romantic Russian music and a Wagnerian flavour gleaned from Lyadov's visit to see Wagner's *Ring Cycle* in St Petersburg in 1889. It was, in fact, these two pieces that persuaded Serge Diaghilev that Lyadov was the man to write his *Firebird* ballet.

Alas, *Zoryushka* never materialized, but Lyadov's music suggests a tantalizing 'what might have been'. He is a composer whose limited output nevertheless placed an influential stamp on Russian music, not least in the music of Alexander Scriabin and Stravinsky, both of whose works owe Lyadov a debt of gratitude. Even Rimsky-Korsakov later regretted expelling Lyadov from the Conservatory, admitting that his pupil had been 'talented past telling' all along.

RECOMMENDED LISTENING

Lyadov – *Ballade (In Olden Days)*
⊙ *Megumi Sano (piano) (ARS Produktion)*

Loneliness

Was Edward Elgar fundamentally lonely? There is evidence that he never settled into Malvern's tranquil pace of life after he and his wife moved back to the Worcestershire town from London in 1891. Bouts of melancholy, flashes of unexpected rudeness and depression dogged him throughout his life. Despite being Britain's most celebrated composer, Elgar never shook off his complex about being the son of a Worcester shopkeeper. Marriage to Alice Roberts had lifted him several rungs up the social ladder, but somehow that made things worse. He loved his wife devotedly, but Elgar never quite felt as though he fitted in with her family. A troubled, often tempestuous seam runs through much of his music, aside from the surface pomp of a few works. The late *Cello Concerto*, his *Symphony No. 1* and the intimate, aching *String Quartet* that was played at Alice's funeral in 1920 are all typical of the composer's reflective spirit.

Among Elgar's happier works, however, is the one that sealed his international reputation. His 1899 *Variations on an Original Theme*, or the *Enigma Variations*, comprises 14 vividly characterized portraits of the sorts of friends we all wish we had: generous, fascinating and hugely amusing. Each intimately crafted orchestral miniature is based on a theme that today remains a mystery, a mischievous detail that perhaps reveals how much Elgar was buoyed up by his friendships.

'Variation I' is a tender tribute to Alice, his former piano pupil who devoted her life to his music. A series of gentle, friendly digs at friends includes the lumbering, whirling 'Variation VII', as Elgar teases his friend Arthur for incompetent piano playing. In 'Variation XI', cascading strings, scampering woodwind, brass fanfares and a final almighty timpani crash capture Hereford Cathedral organist George Sinclair's bulldog, Dan, tumbling down the bank into the River Wye. Not all of Elgar's vignettes are caricatures, however – 'Variation VIII' is the sunniest of them all, an English idyll in music and a tender tribute to musician Winifred Norbury. The most heartfelt variation, the dazzlingly lovely 'Variation IX', called 'Nimrod', is reserved for Elgar's music publisher, Augustus Jaeger, a loyal friend who had helped Elgar through periods of depression, urging him again and again never to forsake composing.

So for half an hour, sit back and revel in the kindness and sparkling company of music's most supportive and close-knit group of friends.

....

Elgar – *Variations on an Original Theme (Enigma Variations)*
◉ *BBC Symphony Orchestra/Andrew Davis (Warner Classics)*

....

Love (unrequited)

With only the rarest of relationships thriving on an equal footing, unrequited love is pain that many of us experience at some point in our lives. Composers' disastrous love lives have produced rich inspiration over the centuries, as the hollow, empty feeling of romantic rejection has shaped some of the most searing and powerful works in the classical canon. If you, too, are cast adrift on the sea of unrequited love, then take comfort in the abundance of music that shares your sorrow.

Like all of us, composers have handled rejection in a variety of ways. Johannes Brahms, whose affections frequently fell on barren ground, poured his heart into music of deep desire. Brahms summed up his feelings for the wife of Robert Schumann, Clara, in the *Piano Quartet No. 3*, its opening marked by sighing falls, musical utterances of 'Clara' that echo throughout the first movement. Brahms and Clara Schumann became close after Robert's death, but as far as we know, Clara – herself a renowned pianist and composer – kept their relationship platonic. A year after Clara's death in 1896, Brahms died, a bachelor to the end.

Other composers dig even deeper into the anguish of heartbreak. Leoš Janáček's obsession with Kamila Stösslová, a married woman 37 years his junior, sparked the creative fire behind the *String Quartet No. 2 'Intimate Letters'*, a reference to the hundreds of times he wrote to her in 1928. The quartet is an inventive, turbulent work, full of imagined erotic passion and nervous expectation, contrasted with jagged indignation and a sense of longing.

There is, however, nothing to rival the sense of the hopelessness of unrequited love in Franz Schubert's *Die schöne Müllerin* ('The Beautiful Maid of the Mill'). By the time Schubert came to compose this great song cycle in 1823, the young Austrian was dying of syphilis, well into a course of mind-altering mercury treatment and in great physical and emotional pain (see also pages 35–6 and 37–8). *Die schöne Müllerin*, setting the words of the poet Wilhelm Müller, charts in 20 songs the journey of a young miller, bathed in contented innocence and delight as he sees a girl and presents her with a green ribbon as a token of his love. A young hunter arrives on the scene to steal the girl away from him, and the miller's mood turns to jealousy and despair. Schubert's powerfully descriptive work follows the contours of the miller's emotions with music that spirals into the depths – such as in 'Trockne Blumen' ('Withered Flowers') – but always remains astonishingly beautiful.

RECOMMENDED LISTENING

Brahms – *Piano Quartet No. 3*
◉ *Artemis Quartet (Erato)*

Janáček – *String Quartet No. 2 'Intimate Letters'*
◉ *Pavel Haas Quartet (Supraphon)*

Schubert – *Die schöne Müllerin*
◉ *Jonas Kaufmann (tenor), Helmut Deutsch (piano) (Decca)*

M

Mental breakdown (understanding)

'Truly there would be a reason to go mad were it not for music', sighed the Russian composer Tchaikovsky, whose music often gave clues to a life lived on an emotional edge. And if music can rescue us from moments of madness, it can also paint brilliant portraits of insanity.

We have seen how the English 17th-century composer Henry Purcell can summon the hollowness of grief and the biting cold of freezing wind (see page 66). In his song 'From Silent Shades', Purcell depicts with equal skill the lovelorn Bess's descent into madness – sorrow contrasted with sudden mad rages ('Did you not see my love') and flashes of almost comic self-pity ('My music shall be a groan').

Half a century later, English artist William Hogarth was chronicling the excesses of 18th-century London in cartoons and paintings, the most famous of which, the series of paintings called *The Rake's Progress*, were adapted for the stage in 1951 by Igor Stravinsky. Hogarth's series charts the decline and fall of the wealthy Tom Rakewell as he succumbs to drink, debauchery and eventual mental breakdown, spending his final days in the city's infamous asylum, Bethlem Hospital. Stravinsky's music, by now in full neo-classical, almost Mozartian bloom (a far cry from *The Rite of Spring*; see page 131), depicts Tom's tragic descent into mental collapse with striking sparseness and simplicity.

In total contrast, the mad scene from Gaetano Donizetti's opera *Lucia di Lammermoor* features a series of technically demanding arias (including the beautiful 'Il dolce suono') that stretch the lead soprano's technical abilities to their limits. Driven mad (and eventually to her grave) by the machinations of the various men in her life, Lucia acts out her mental crisis in vocal acrobatics that the great sopranos, including Joan Sutherland, have embellished with trills, scales and ornamentation, making them even more difficult – and madder – than Donizetti necessarily intended. Perhaps the greatest and dramatically most accomplished soprano of them all, Maria Callas, caused a scandal in opera circles in 1955 by performing the scene *come scritto* ('as written') – proving that even in madness, less is more.

RECOMMENDED LISTENING

Purcell – *From Silent Shades*
⊙ *Stéphanie d'Oustrac (mezzo), Ensemble Amarillis/Héloïse Gaillard (Harmonia Mundi)*

Stravinsky – *The Rake's Progress*
⊙ *Ian Bostridge, Bryn Terfel and more, Monteverdi Choir, London Symphony Orchestra/ John Eliot Gardiner (Deutsche Grammophon)*

Donizetti – *Lucia di Lammermoor*
⊙ *Maria Callas (soprano), Chorus and Orchestra of the Maggio Musicale Fiorentino/ Tullio Serafin (Naxos)*

M

Mirth (lack of)

It is well proven that music can cheer us up, but we are unlikely to go to a concert or head to our record collection if we are in need of a good laugh, saving that job for films, TV, books, poetry, theatre and, naturally, live comedy. Classical music is full of pieces that raise a smile, a muted snort at most, but there are a few funny ones nevertheless. Here are three of the best.

Long attributed to Haydn but now known to be the work of Wolfgang Amadeus Mozart's father, Leopold, the *Toy Symphony* is scored for orchestra and an assembly of toy instruments, including drum, cuckoo, nightingale, rattle and triangle. Delivery here is the key, and the piece is best seen live and performed straight. The comedy comes mostly from the sight of adult musicians grappling with a battery of tiny instruments against the unexceptional, four-square orchestral accompaniment.

The *Duetto Buffo di Due Gatti* ('Cat Duet'), attributed to Gioachino Rossini but probably by English composer Robert Pearsall, unites two rival cats, played by a couple of meowing sopranos. Written in the style of an Italian opera aria, the piece leaves ample room for the singers to place their own character on each cat. But beware the soprano who tries too hard – in the wrong hands, this exquisitely funny piece can quickly descend into an embarrassing mess. The trick is to use two sopranos best known for serious opera roles. Then the Cat Duet is a hilarious delight.

The comic crown, however, goes to Malcolm Arnold, a composer with an almost endless stylistic range. *A Grand, Grand Overture* was written in 1956 for one of a series of concerts organized by Arnold's friend the artist, musician and humorist Gerard Hoffnung, and is scored for orchestra, organ, three vacuum cleaners, one electric floor polisher and four rifles. It is dedicated to the American President Herbert Hoover and employs just about every musical weapon in Arnold's armoury, from whimsical to grand ceremonial. The gorgeous opening string chords and fluttering piccolo suggest a work of serious intent – but then the floor polishers start up. Arnold's final comic flourish is to send himself up – four marksmen appear and take aim at each of the floor-cleaning soloists. Perfectly executed comedy.

RECOMMENDED LISTENING

Mozart (Leopold) – *Toy Symphony*
⊙ *I Musici de Montréal/Yuli Turovsky (Chandos)*

Attributed to Rossini – *Duetto Buffo di Due Gatti*
⊙ *Victoria de los Ángeles (soprano), Elisabeth Schwarzkopf (soprano), Gerald Moore (piano) (Warner Classics)*

M

Arnold – *A Grand, Grand Overture*
⊙ *Royal Philharmonic Orchestra/Vernon Handley (Sony)*

Moodiness

It was the summer of 1830, and Felix Mendelssohn was feeling great. The talented 21-year-old German composer had already packed a lot into his life, dashing off a vast amount of music in youthful, white-hot inspiration. His *Symphony No. 1*, the incidental music to Shakespeare's *A Midsummer Night's Dream* and a dazzling *String Octet* (see page 16) joined a host of other brilliant works. The previous year had been especially busy. In March 1829, Mendelssohn had conducted the first performance of Johann Sebastian Bach's *St Matthew Passion* since the composer's death in 1750, and just a month later had embarked on a tour of Britain, giving performances in London as both a conductor and a pianist. Walking holidays in Wales and Scotland followed, before he boarded a boat to the Outer Hebrides, where, between bouts of seasickness, he sketched what would turn out to be his most famous orchestral work, *The Hebrides Overture* (see page 129). Now it was time for a holiday. His destination was Italy, with Venice, Florence, Rome, Genoa, Naples and Milan all firmly in his sights.

Mendelssohn kept a record of his Grand Tour in a set of accomplished watercolours of the Amalfi coast, diary entries of almost breathless excitement and joyful letters home. One of them, to his mother, spoke of a new orchestral work, inspired by the architecture, countryside and people he encountered on his way. 'I have once more begun to compose with fresh vigour, and the Italian symphony makes rapid progress,' he wrote. 'It will be the most joyful thing I have yet composed.' This symphony (his *Symphony No. 4*) stayed in Mendelssohn's head until his return to Berlin in 1832, whereupon London's Royal Philharmonic Society offered him a symphonic commission, and the music flowed.

True to his word, the symphony's opening movement is pure Mediterranean sun, with a first-movement melody that leaps and skips and laughs. Even its churchly second movement wears an air of contentment, while the finale, the mischievous 'Saltarello', bursts with energy and a zest for life. It is a sparkling portrait of the Italian spirit and of a carefree young adult. It is classical music at its happiest – the perfect antidote to moodiness.

RECOMMENDED LISTENING

Mendelssohn – *Symphony No. 4 ('Italian')*
⊙ *City of Birmingham Symphony Orchestra/Edward Gardner (Chandos)*

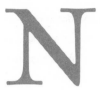

Nastiness

Composers write music to describe the full range of emotions and situations – and that sometimes means the nastiest, goriest, most violent ones imaginable. After all, classical music is not short of gruesome stories, being full of beheadings, stabbings, self-disembowelment and even cannibalism. It is a rare composer who can craft a score of stomach-churning horrors – most only manage some sort of ominous mood music. But there are some who can paint the most abhorrent pictures in just a few bars, bringing the unimaginable to spectacularly gory sonic life.

So, hopefully, you'll find that your own troubles with nastiness pale in comparison to the spiteful misdemeanours of old – if your crimes go further than those explored in the classical canon I fear you may beyond the reach of this book. With that in mind, here are the finest examples of the most sickening music ever written. A quintet of masterpieces with the power to bring even the nastiest of you to your senses.

Strauss – *Salome*

Richard Strauss's 1905 opera contains a scene in which the severed head of John the Baptist is brought out on a platter, whereupon Salome kisses it passionately on the lips before being crushed to death on the orders of Herod. Strauss responds with incredible music that combines a post-Romantic richness with bursts of almost overwhelming atonality.

⊙ *Malin Byström, Doris Soffel, Evgeny Nikitin, Royal Concertgebouw Orchestra/Daniele Gatti (RCO Live)*

Bartók – *The Miraculous Mandarin Suite*

Another horrific plot, this time by Béla Bartók, telling the story of a girl who lures passersby into her room to be robbed by her accomplices. Among them is a Chinese man who, when attacked, refuses to die. Only when the girl satisfies his desire does he finally succumb to his wounds. The opening claustrophobic music and final frenzied bars, complete with jagged rhythms and *glissando* brass, are shocking and nightmarish.

⊙ *Helsinki Philharmonic Orchestra/Susanna Mälkki (BIS)*

Poulenc – *Dialogues of the Carmelites*

Francis Poulenc's operatic telling of the execution of an order of nuns during the French Revolution juxtaposes a soaring, defiant chorus with the sickening thuds of a guillotine as each nun walks up the scaffold. Poulenc's masterly blend of music and effects, with the right sound balance, never fails to turn the stomach.

⊙ *Opéra National de Lyon, Chorus of the Opéra National de Lyon/Kent Nagano (Erato)*

Benjamin – *Written on Skin*

At the end of George Benjamin's acclaimed 2013 psychological opera, The Protector cooks Agnès a meal, which she eats and enjoys, later learning that it included the heart of a young boy. Benjamin sizes up to the challenges of this horrendous scene with music that blends a disturbing intimacy with blood-curdling musical eruptions.

⊙ *Christopher Purves, Barbara Hannigan, Bejun Mehta, Mahler Chamber Orchestra/ George Benjamin (Nimbus)*

Crumb – *Black Angels*

American composer George Crumb's 1971 work for electric string quartet, 'a kind of parable on our troubled contemporary world', according to the composer, begins with a terrifying and unsettling evocation of the attack helicopters used by the US army during the Vietnam War. Crumb's instruction for the work's volume to be increased 'to the threshold of pain' only adds to its horror.

⊙ *Kronos Quartet (Nonesuch)*

Naughtiness (in adults)

What does the word 'naughty' mean to you? If we are talking about basic bad behaviour, then classical music has no shortage of composers who really should have known better. In fact, it may be surprising to learn, given the calibre of the music they produced, just how badly behaved some of them were. Debussy, Delius, Wagner and Bax all wandered outside their marriages (Arnold Bax is famous for his suggestion that everyone should try everything once, except morris dancing and incest), while Sibelius, though loyal, referred to alcohol rather than his wife as 'his most faithful companion' – it was his long-suffering wife, Aino, who would regularly drag him home from Helsinki's bars.

On the other hand, there is a side to adult naughtiness that suggests something a little more light-hearted – saucy, even. To access that kind of, arguably more harmless, naughtiness, the soundtracks to the *Carry On* films have never been bettered. Tapping into the traditions of early-20th-century music halls, the British *Carry On* films of the 1960s and '70s were packed full of irreverent humour, with a roster of cast members who stayed with the 31-film series throughout, including Kenneth Williams, Barbara Windsor, Charles Hawtrey, Sid James and Joan Sims. Send-ups of the police force, camping holidays, the National Health Service, the British army and many more were done with a combination of sexual innuendo and slapstick humour.

None of those films would be nearly as funny if it were not for the vivid soundtracks that brought their naughtiness to life. The 31 soundtracks were written by just two composers, Bruce Montgomery (also a crime writer and the composer of the original *Carry On* theme) and Eric Rogers (who orchestrated the original stage production of Lionel Bart's musical *Oliver!*). Together, their music was brilliantly and often grandly orchestrated, each score parading a perkiness that combines Big Band jazz with a cartoonlike character, all bundled up in British swagger. For a taste of many of the naughty *Carry On* vibes, seek out the *Carry On Suite*, which was arranged by David Whittle from the scores of *Carry On Sergeant*, *Carry On Teacher* and *Carry On Nurse*.

RECOMMENDED LISTENING

Montgomery – *Carry On Suite*
⊙ *City of Prague Philharmonic/Gavin Sutherland (White Line)*

Nostalgia (excessive)

Richard Strauss was one of the greatest composers of the late 19th and early 20th centuries, a man with an unrivalled talent for melody and orchestration. By the time he died in 1949, aged 85, the world had been technologically, politically and culturally transformed, while two world wars had devastated Europe and humiliated Strauss's German homeland. From his first major work, the 1880

Symphony No. 1, his music veered between solid conservatism and the shocking modernism of, say, his 1909 opera *Elektra*. Among the composer's greatest music, however, are dozens of Romantic songs for soprano and orchestra written for and inspired by his wife, the soprano Pauline de Ahna. And it is to the orchestral song that Strauss turned for his final works – four incredible, richly scored jewels written in 1948, later gathered together and published as the *Four Last Songs*.

Among the most exquisite music of anything written in the 20th century, the *Four Last Songs* combine wistful glances to a pre-War age with a gentle acceptance of death. In the first three songs, setting poems by Hermann Hesse, Strauss takes the listener from the promise of spring ('the world sparkles in the light of a miracle') through to autumn, when summer departs, the garden mourns and 'the flowers fill with cold rain'. For the final song, a setting of 'At Sunset' by Joseph von Eichendorff, Strauss conjures a magical image of an elderly couple watching the sunset, looking back on their lives and finding beauty in their final moments. Strauss accompanies their journey with sumptuous string writing, lingering vocal lines and, to finish, fluttering lark song that soars over gentle shifts between minor and major towards the final, peaceful chord. As the orchestra fades into the distance, there is a sense that Strauss is not simply bidding farewell to his own life, but also to the Romantic musical tradition he held dear throughout his career.

As we grow older and look back on our lives, Strauss's music is a powerful reminder to find inner peace and to put our regrets behind us.

RECOMMENDED LISTENING

Strauss – *Four Last Songs*
◉ *Soile Isokoski (soprano), Berlin Radio Symphony Orchestra/Marek Janowski (Pentatone)*

O

Obsession

We all have our obsessions. It might be a soap opera, say, or dusting every corner of the house. Football might occupy your every waking thought, or that perfect golf swing you dream about every night. For Baroque composer Johann Sebastian Bach, it was the fugue. Throughout his life, Bach composed music in every musical form, for every musical instrument. Sonatas, concertos, cantatas, masses, preludes, partitas, toccatas and more all formed part of Bach's incredible output of over 1,000 works. Yet the fugue was the one musical form that dominated everything else. Put simply, a fugue is characterized by a principal theme or 'subject' that repeats and combines in different forms and keys – a complex mathematical piece and yet, in the right hands, something satisfying and mesmerizing.

You will find fugues everywhere in Bach's music – in the *Brandenburg Concertos*, in the cello suites, orchestral suites and, naturally, in the preludes and fugues that make up Books 1 and 2 of *The Well-Tempered Clavier* and much of his music for the pipe organ. Towards the end of his life, Bach was living in a world that was fast transitioning from the complex age of the Baroque to the clearer, simpler, more melodic Classical era typified by Haydn and Mozart. This meant that the fugue would soon become a rare beast. The more the Classical style spread across the Western musical world, the tighter Bach held onto the fugue.

At his death, Bach left unfinished his ultimate fugal statement, the theoretical *The Art of Fugue*; in it the form is taken to its natural conclusion, its 14 fugues (and 4 canons) arranged in order of increasing complexity. Composed for unspecified instruments, but most commonly performed today on keyboard or by a string quartet, *The Art of Fugue* is based on a single theme that is inverted, mirrored, augmented, diminished and placed in among double and triple fugues (in which the fugue has two or three themes running concurrently). The collection includes an unfinished four-voice triple fugue that incorporates the letters BACH, corresponding to the German names for the notes B flat, A, C and B natural. Did Bach leave this breathtaking fugue incomplete due to failing sight, or as a challenge for others to take up the mantle?

If you have an obsessive nature, Bach's music is proof that it can lead to great personal riches – you just need to steer it in the right direction.

RECOMMENDED LISTENING

Bach – *The Art of Fugue*
⊙ *Grigory Sokolov (piano) (Naïve)*

Overstimulation

Music is almost always the right response to life's ills, but when the world seems a little too full of noises, when listening to music simply substitutes sound for another sound, then music is not the answer – not in the conventional sense, anyway.

John Cage originally dreamed up *4'33"* in the late 1940s as an antidote to life's incessant soundtrack. In a lecture, he had suggested sending a recording of silence to Muzak, a company responsible for the background music in shops, restaurants and other public spaces. But a visit in 1951 to an anechoic chamber that completely absorbed all sound revealed to him that silence was impossible: in a room purporting to be silent, Cage could still hear the sounds of his nervous system and his circulating blood.

So *4'33"* was composed not as a piece of anti-music, or a gimmick, but as a way to bring us back to ourselves and make us aware of our surroundings. As the pianist David Tudor said after the premiere of the work at the Maverick Concert Hall near Woodstock, in New York state, *4'33"* was 'one of the most intense listening experiences you can have'.

But is it classical music? There is a strong argument that suggests it is, that Cage's piece only really works in the traditional environment of a classical music concert, in an auditorium where people are used to being silent for unusually long periods of time but where there is plenty of ambient noise – rustling programmes, stifled coughs, squeaking chairs, heavy breathing. On the other hand, why should *4'33"* not be enjoyed by an audience of one, in the comfort of their own home? In fact, why should you not perform it yourself, at the same time as listening to it? After all, Cage specified that his work 'may be performed by any instrumentalist or combination of instrumentalists'. And he did not stipulate how good you need to be at that instrument, nor did he say how closely you had to listen to your ambient sounds.

Whether it is classical or not does not really matter. *4'33"* lets you indulge, as performer and listener, in a modernist masterpiece, while giving you a chance to switch off for a while.

RECOMMENDED LISTENING

....

Cage – *4'33"*
⊙ *Performed by you!*

....

P

Panic

A sudden panic episode can be frightening, as it may appear as if from nowhere. One of the tragedies of modern life is that too many of us parade our hectic, relentless lives as if they were badges of honour. Full-time jobs creep into extra time, children have to be brought up, friendships need to be maintained, professional relationships must be nurtured. Take your eyes off low-lying anxiety and it can easily morph into panic. Of course, panic can be caused by many things, including sudden emotional shocks such as bereavement, or, physiologically, by an imbalance of neurotransmitters in the brain. It may be that a predisposition to feelings of panic runs in the family. As with any serious condition, it is crucial that sufferers seek medical help as soon as possible – treatments can range from sessions of cognitive behavioural therapy to breathing exercises to activities such as yoga and pilates.

Music can also help to calm and relax, but while a piece of music may appear to be soothing at the outset, more than likely it fluctuates in its general mood and dynamics. Here, however, are five works that maintain their levels of calm, guaranteeing you space to stop and breathe.

Einaudi – *Seven Days Walking*
In 2018, the Italian pianist and composer Ludovico Einaudi made a series of

walks in the Alps, 'always following more or less the same trail'. The result, a year later, was a series of gentle, hypnotic albums, *Seven Days Walking*, scored for piano and strings.

⊙ *Ludovico Einaudi (piano) (Decca)*

Morricone – 'Gabriel's Oboe' from *The Mission*

England rugby captain Will Carling once admitted on BBC Radio 4's *Desert Island Discs* programme that he would listen to this beautiful tune from Ennio Morricone's Oscar-nominated soundtrack to instil in him a sense of calm before an international match.

⊙ *Ennio Morricone and His Orchestra (Deutsche Grammophon)*

Lloyd Webber – *Invocation*

William Lloyd Webber (Andrew Lloyd Webber's father) was a celebrated orchestral and choral composer, as well as a respected organist and choral director. This exquisite piece for strings, harp and timpani is a *bona fide* miniature masterpiece.

⊙ *City of London Sinfonia/Richard Hickox (Chandos)*

Shostakovich – 'Andante' from *Piano Concerto No. 2*

Dmitri Shostakovich wrote this piano concerto for his son, Maxim, to perform. It features one of his most magical slow movements, devoid of any of the angst that troubles much of his music.

⊙ *Dmitri Alexeev (piano), English Chamber Orchestra/Jerzy Maksymiuk (Warner Classics)*

Debussy – *Arabesque No. 1*

One of the French Impressionist composer Claude Debussy's early piano works, the rippling *Arabesque* has a beautiful simplicity, with flowing melodic lines and timeless modal harmonies that evoke balmy summer evenings on the Seine.

⊙ *Jean-Yves Thibaudet (piano) (Decca)*

....

Passion (lack of)

'Never compose anything unless the not composing of it becomes a positive nuisance to you.' Gustav Holst's quote from a letter to a friend perfectly sums up the driving nature of passion. A passion for something or someone is an unstoppable force, a feeling that nothing else matters, even your own well-being. No wonder: the word derives from the Latin *passio*, meaning to suffer or endure. Passion is what has driven writers, artists, poets and composers through the ages to forgo financial security in pursuit of spiritual fulfilment. It drives us to achieve greatness no matter what, to be our very best. But it is also a privilege that not all of us experience in our lives. Not everyone has dreams, and even those who do often end up ignoring them.

Behind success, particularly artistic success, are hard work, determination and self-sacrifice. It is easy to forget that many of the great composers never really 'made it'. Mozart died penniless, Beethoven was once so angered over the loss of a penny that he wrote a piece about it (see page 68), and Holst was at one time so poor that he had to walk the 160km (100 miles) from London, where he was studying, to his Cheltenham home. Even Puccini, famed for his high living in later life, once wrote to his mother from Milan: 'I'm not starving, but I wouldn't say I'm eating well. I fill up with minestrone, thin broth and still thinner broth.'

If you are still searching for your life's passion, do not give up. You may well find it tomorrow, you may discover it in your eighties. Until then, be inspired by

P

the quirky piano works of Erik Satie, Paris's iconic 20th-century practitioner of Surrealism and Dada, who lived in a grimy flat in the Paris suburbs and subsidized his life as a 'serious' composer by playing in cafés and writing cabaret music. You do not have to be rich to be famous – but you do have to be passionate.

RECOMMENDED LISTENING

Satie – *Gymnopédie No. 1*
◉ *Pascal Rogé (piano) (Decca)*

Peril

In addition to the all-important schmaltzy love theme, film composers usually count 'menace' among the most important musical tools in their kitbag. John Williams's opening theme to the 1975 film *Jaws* is a case in point. Its initial two-note motif, angular French horn countermelodies and, at the point of the first shark attack, swirling, screeching strings and stabbing percussion are terrifying. Bernard Hermann was arguably the master of menace, which explains why he was the composer of choice for film director Alfred Hitchcock. Hermann, Williams and others, however, took their cues from a variety of classical works that brilliantly convey atmospheres of threat and peril. The five works below may not make for pleasant listening, but they'll place your own feelings of peril in perspective and may even banish them for good.

Scriabin – *Piano Sonata No. 9 'Black Mass'*
Alexander Scriabin's disconcerting one-movement sonata, dating from around 1913, grows in intensity from its sinister opening to a raging march-like climax.

In the final minutes, the opening returns once again, creeping towards an uncertain, unresolved conclusion.

⊙ *Yevgeny Sudbin (piano) (BIS)*

....

Mussorgsky – *A Night on Bald Mountain*

Right from the start, Modest Mussorgsky's sole tone poem (adapted by Rimsky-Korsakov) whips up a wild, stormy atmosphere, its depiction of a witches' sabbath on a mountain near Kiev full of chromatic harmonies, sudden furious bursts of sound and menacing rhythms.

⊙ *Mariinsky Orchestra/Valery Gergiev (Mariinsky)*

....

Liszt – *Totentanz*

Franz Liszt's 'dance of death', inspired by medieval depictions of death, gets its sense of looming terror from the pounding chromatic piano chords that dominate the opening bars, sudden eruptions from the orchestra, and Liszt's use of the spooky Gregorian 'Dies irae' chant theme.

⊙ *Louis Lortie (piano), The Hague Philharmonic Orchestra/George Pehlivanian (Chandos)*

....

Britten – 'Storm' from *Four Sea Interludes*

It is not so much a literal storm that Benjamin Britten is describing in this interlude from the opera *Peter Grimes*, but the threat and menace of a local community, determined to wreak misdirected revenge on a fisherman they accuse of murdering his apprentice.

⊙ *Orchestra of the Royal Opera House Covent Garden/Benjamin Britten (Decca)*

....

Ravel – *Gaspard de la nuit*

Maurice Ravel's piano suite contains one of the most challenging movements in the whole piano repertoire, and one of its most menacing. 'Scarbo' depicts the wild flight of a goblin in terrifying, macabre music that skits in and out of the shadows.

⊙ *Steven Osborne (piano) (Hyperion)*

....

Pessimism

From the daring, glorious vulgarity of its opening clarinet *glissando* to its infectious blues melodies and thumping syncopations, George Gershwin's *Rhapsody in Blue* screams optimism, making it the perfect antidote to a case of excessive negativity. The United States in the 1920s was a nation full of hope and confidence. The First World War was behind it, the Spanish flu had all but petered out, and the economy was at an all-time high. Never mind the imminent Wall Street Crash or the Great Depression – before all that, the US was celebrating. Classical music was too serious to match the party mood. What it needed was an injection of jazz and a respected composer who could sneak its 'commotion without repose' into the concert hall. That the French, including the likes of Satie and Debussy, had already been toying with jazz for some years was quietly forgotten as the US became the centre of musical innovation.

In 1924 Gershwin was invited by the great jazz band leader Paul Whiteman to write a piece for piano and 23-man band, to be performed at New York's Aeolian Hall with the composer himself as soloist. The skeleton score for *Rhapsody in Blue* was completed in a white-hot three-week frenzy, and orchestrated in just ten days by composer and arranger Ferde Grofé. It was not an instant hit – it was described by one critic as 'derivative..., stale... and so inexpressive' – but it did not matter. The piece, the rhythms of which were inspired, according to the composer himself, by the movement and noise of the New York–Boston commuter train, was a blast of fresh air. Liszt and Chopin blended with ragtime and African-American blues, along with smatterings of Debussy, whose exotic, sultry music had already pushed the harmonic envelope since the turn of the 20th century. Classical music would never be quite the same again. As a symbol of America's buoyant mood, and as a great turning point in its music culture, *Rhapsody in Blue* has never been matched.

RECOMMENDED LISTENING

Gershwin – *Rhapsody in Blue*
⊙ *André Previn (piano), London Symphony Orchestra/André Previn (Warner Classics)*

Pettiness

It would be fantastic if everyone just relaxed a bit and realized that we are all trying to do our best. When we have our priorities wrong, or are feeling too self-important, pettiness can set in. Pettiness is the committee secretary sticking to arcane meeting rules, or the middle manager a little lacking in people skills. And it can afflict even the greatest of conductors. A petty conductor likes nothing better than to call out a wrong note in the horn section – and to make the offending musician practise out the error in front of everyone.

Maestro Colin Davis had a reputation as a young man for shouting at and verbally abusing his musicians in rehearsal, with one calling him 'a very difficult man to like'. The nadir perhaps came in 1973, when his productions of Beethoven's *Fidelio*, Wagner's *Tannhäuser* and Mozart's *Don Giovanni* were booed at London's Covent Garden. His reaction? To stick his tongue out at the audience and boo them back.

But Davis's temper tantrums were nothing compared to those of the fearsome Italian maestro Arturo Toscanini, who took pettiness to a whole new level, insulting members of the orchestra and, according to Samuel Antek's entertaining book *This Was Toscanini*, ripping his own jacket to shreds in exasperation. On one occasion, a member of the NBC Symphony Orchestra dared answer back, explaining that a demand from Toscanini to play *piano* should, in fact, be *forte*. Antek's account of the episode is fascinating:

> What means 'forte'? Ignorante! Is a stupid word — as stupid as you! Is a thousand fortes — all kinds of fortes. Sometimes forte is *pia-a-a-no*, *piano* is *forte*! *Accidenti!* [Damn it!] You call yourself a musician? *O, per Dio santissimo!* You play here in *this* orchestra? In a village café house you belong!

At least Toscanini did not go on stage with a loaded pistol in his jacket pocket, as did the American-Polish conductor Artur Rodzinski. Rumour had it that Rodzinski carried the pistol as a good luck charm, having once given a particularly fine performance before which he had forgotten to remove the weapon from his person.

Perhaps, however, we should learn from the great Leonard Bernstein, a master of self-control. In a filmed rehearsal of Elgar's *Enigma Variations* with the BBC Symphony Orchestra, the American conductor, composer and educator tries to tell the trumpet section how to shape a particular phrase while giving it a more rounded tone. One of the three trumpeters tests Bernstein by answering back, but the clearly exhausted conductor replies with a blithe 'Well, that's strange...' and shames him into a perfect performance.

Listen to the fiery opening movement of Gustav Mahler's *Symphony No. 5*, recorded in 1967 by the New York Philharmonic under Bernstein. Marvel at the magnificent, epic music — but also at how much can be achieved if we keep everything a little more in perspective.

RECOMMENDED LISTENING

Mahler – *Symphony No. 5*

⊙ *New York Philharmonic/Leonard Bernstein (Sony Classical)*

Procrastination

Chances are you may be reading this when you should be washing the dishes, mowing the lawn or taking the dog for its daily walk. You then might pick up your phone and pointlessly scroll through social media for a couple of hours. Before you know it, someone else has gathered your socks and tidied up around you. Even the great composers were not immune to procrastination.

It is hard to believe that the composer of almost 40 operas could be anything other than expert at time management, but Gioachino Rossini had an irritating habit of leaving things to the last minute. The fact that he wrote the entire score of *The Barber of Seville* in 13 days is not, in fact, the sign of a highly productive man, but of someone whose favourite sound was the whoosh of deadlines passing by. Even Hector Berlioz saw through Rossini's working habits, accusing him of cutting corners with an 'endless repetition of a single form of cadence'.

A newspaper report from 1897 describes Rossini's last-minute dash to write the overture to *The Thieving Magpie*, an opera about a young girl falsely accused of stealing. 'The overture to the "Gazza Ladra" [*Thieving Magpie*] was written under curious circumstances,' observed the weekly newspaper *Ann Arbor Argus* from Michigan, in the United States:

> On the very day of the first performance of the opera, not a note of the overture was written, and the manager, getting hold of Rossini, confined

P

him in the upper loft of La Scala, setting four scene-shifters on guard over him. These took the sheets as they were filled and threw them out of the windows to copyists beneath.

But the opera's overture was one of Rossini's finest creations, with bold use of snare drum (later heard accompanying the accused's march to the scaffold) and a magnificent military march that sets the scene for the hero Giannetto's jubilant return from the war. It is also one of the most frequently performed of Rossini's works and a reminder that dithering can, in fact, often go hand-in-hand with inspiration.

RECOMMENDED LISTENING

Rossini – 'Overture' from *The Thieving Magpie*
◉ *London Symphony Orchestra/Claudio Abbado (Deutsche Grammophon)*

P

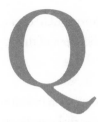

Queasiness

Those with children know that long car journeys are guaranteed to be accompanied by two things: constant queries of 'Are we nearly there yet?', asked with varying degrees of disappointment and desperation, and car sickness. The music that makes people feel queasy is often the piece they listened to most in the car on the way to family holidays or trips to see Granny. It might be The Beatles' *Sgt. Pepper's Lonely Hearts Club Band*, Saint-Saëns's piano concertos or a Bach *Brandenburg Concerto* – even music far removed from any notion of queasiness can bring you straight back to that feeling of nausea that we all felt as the highway spooled out to the soundtrack of our childhoods. One imperfect remedy, arguably, is to steer clear of these works.

Decades before cars, it was a sea journey that made Felix Mendelssohn so seasick that he could not even come above deck to visit Staffa, a remote, rocky outcrop of basalt in the Outer Hebrides, under which lurks Fingal's Cave. Mendelssohn's *The Hebrides Overture*, nicknamed 'Fingal's Cave', brings the swelling sea and rocking boat to queasy life from the opening bar, with an ingenious motif played by the string section and a use of rapid *crescendos* and *diminuendos* (see also page 109).

György Ligeti's *Etude No. 9* for solo piano, called 'Vertige' ('Dizziness'), is a dizzying, disorientating listen that uses overlapping chromatic scales to create the illusion of an endless falling movement. It is also one of the most challenging of the Hungarian composer's works for piano, with the composer instructing the pianist to play as fast possible, *legato*, *pianissimo* – and all without using the sustain pedal. It is enough to make even the performer feel a little sick.

Finally, although British composer Anna Clyne's *Night Ferry* is a 20-minute work for orchestra intended principally to portray the rapid shifts between mental states from which Robert Schumann acutely suffered (see pages 35–6), it is also a swirling, multi-layered piece that, like Mendelssohn's *Fingal's Cave,* takes us far from shore.

As with seasickness itself, the way to combat queasiness is to exercise a little mind over matter. Listen to these works several times, and you'll find yourself growing steadily immune to their effects.

RECOMMENDED LISTENING

Mendelssohn – *The Hebrides Overture ('Fingal's Cave')*
⊙ *London Symphony Orchestra/John Eliot Gardiner (LSO Live)*

Clyne – *Night Ferry*
⊙ *BBC Symphony Orchestra/Andrew Litton (Avie)*

Ligeti – *Etude No. 9 ('Vertige')*
⊙ *Danny Driver (piano) (Hyperion)*

R

Rebelliousness

Conforming is comfortable, but you cannot be a genius without a streak of rebelliousness. Our lives have been revolutionized by people who have swum against the tide: Einstein, Turing, Picasso, Shakespeare – and Igor Stravinsky, a man who as a child saw Tchaikovsky conduct in St Petersburg, and who died a year after The Beatles had disbanded.

Over the centuries there have been composers who have challenged the norm: Berlioz, with his eccentric notions of orchestra texture; Beethoven, with musical ideas that stretched far beyond his era; Wagner, a man whose operas took musical drama to daring new heights. But Stravinsky changed the world with just one work, a ballet score so fundamentally different from all that had come before that its 1913 Paris premiere provoked a riot among the audience. Far from destroying the Russian composer's career, *The Rite of Spring* turned him into an overnight sensation, even if none of his subsequent works were quite as controversial.

Depicting a series of primitive rituals, including the sacrifice of a young girl who dances herself to death, *The Rite of Spring*'s savagely discordant music, snarling, crashing chords and constant, unpredictable changes in time signature would have been provocative wherever it was premiered. In refined pre-First-World-War Paris, it created utter havoc. Audience murmuring started just a few bars into the introduction, and before long catcalls and shouting drowned out the music. The dancing did not help. Choreographed by Vaslav Nijinsky for impresario Serge Diaghilev's Ballets Russes, *The Rite of Spring* was as far from a traditional ballet production as one could get. Instead of ballerinas in tutus, the curtain rose to, in Stravinsky's own words, 'a row of braided and knock-kneed Lolitas jumping up and down'.

More than a century after its notorious first performance, Stravinsky's ballet feels both modern and ancient, its primitive rhythms and Russian folk songs placed within startlingly creative and pioneering orchestration. The blood-curdling, dissonant final chord that kills the girl still feels shocking. After its eventful premiere, Stravinsky, Diaghilev and Nijinsky reportedly retired to a quiet dinner, congratulating themselves on a job well done. Stravinsky's musical rebellion had helped shake France's music scene to its roots. You're not being rebellious – you're changing perceptions. Stravinsky's *Rite of Spring* will convince you of that.

RECOMMENDED LISTENING

Stravinsky – *The Rite of Spring*
⊙ *MusicAeterna/Teodor Currentzis (Sony)*

R

Regret

In the summer of 1803, Ludwig van Beethoven rented a house in the village of Oberdöbling, near Heiligenstadt, just to the north of Vienna. He knew Heiligenstadt well – just eight months previously, the 31-year-old German composer had sketched out his devastating Heiligenstadt Testament there, a letter to his brothers that described his horror in the face of his increasing deafness. The act of documenting his personal crisis jolted him from the inside, and the following months became something of a creative turning point, his music exploding with new ideas and bursting with humanity. Oberdöbling became the place where his Third Symphony, the 'Eroica', was born.

The symphony's subject matter would prove the perfect expression of his new-found creative spark. Napoleon Bonaparte was, in Beethoven's eyes, the liberator of Europe, the man who could bring an end to tyranny and usher in republican governments, finally bringing peace to the continent. His 'Bonaparte' Symphony, as he initially called it, would paint a picture of his hero's life in epic fashion, as a way to beckon the revolutionary spirit eastwards towards Germany.

The first movement of the 'Eroica' opens with primal chords, its dissonances, rhythmic confusion, energy and bombast describing Napoleon's struggles on the battlefield. The second movement, a funeral march, sees the composer weeping as he looks to the future and imagines the death of his hero, gazing on the coffin as it is processed through the streets. The third movement, a triumphant 'Scherzo', dances in defiance of death, and the finale features a set of variations on a theme Beethoven had previously used for his ballet, *The Creatures of Prometheus*. For the composer, Prometheus represented Napoleon: a man who had incurred the gods' wrath, taken risks and suffered in order to rescue his comrades.

In 1804, however, as Beethoven was completing his great work, Napoleon declared himself emperor – arguably a tyrant in all but name. Beethoven was appalled and instantly regretted the personal tribute. 'Is he too, then, nothing more than an ordinary human being?' he spluttered. 'Now he, too, will trample on the rights of man, and indulge only his ambition!' Beethoven took the score of his symphony and scrubbed out his dedication to Napoleon so hard that he left a hole in the paper. The 'Bonaparte' Symphony was transformed into the 'Eroica' – a work to the memory of a great man.

Perhaps the antidote to regret is fresh hope? A blast of the symphony's opening movement may help you move past regret and look to a brighter future.

RECOMMENDED LISTENING

Beethoven – *Symphony No. 3 'Eroica'*
⊙ *Berlin Philharmonic/Claudio Abbado (Deutsche Grammophon)*

Rejection

In the spring of 1968, the American film composer Alex North strolled into the New York premiere of Stanley Kubrick's science fiction film *2001: A Space Odyssey*. Kubrick had hired North the previous year on the back of his Oscar-winning score for *Spartacus*, also directed by Kubrick, and the composer had worked day and night in a rented London apartment to meet the director's tight deadlines. Struggling through muscle spasms and back ache, North composed 40 minutes of music in just two weeks and arrived at the recording studio in an ambulance. Kubrick had not told him that he had no intention of using his music, having already decided instead to keep *2001*'s 'temp' tracks – pieces of music that directors often used as place holders while an original soundtrack was being prepared. Alarm bells should have rung when Kubrick commissioned North by playing various records down the phone, asking him to match them for style and mood, while suggesting that North's music would only be one aspect of the final soundtrack.

So as North took his seat in New York's Capitol Theatre and listened with anticipation for his dramatic opening music, what he actually heard was the introduction to Richard Strauss's 1896 tone poem, *Also Sprach Zarathustra*. As the film progressed, North was faced with the agonizing reality that every brilliant note of his had been replaced with music by Johann Strauss II, György Ligeti and Aram Khachaturian. Only now did he realize that his music had been sidelined. Kubrick, famously tricky to work with, had simply not bothered to tell him. This was not just a cruel rejection – it was more akin to a humiliating public drubbing by social media.

North's soundtrack was eventually released in 1993 – and you can hear where he tried to match Kubrick's vision. His introduction has the grandeur of *Also Sprach Zarathustra*, complete with its ominous opening drone, brass fanfare and pipe organ that, like the Strauss, holds on after the orchestra comes off. Where Kubrick substitutes *The Blue Danube* waltz, North's music dances and scampers, gorgeous string *glissandos* lending it a slightly gaudy 1960s sheen. In hindsight, Kubrick was probably right to go with his instinct, but he was clearly a terrible people manager.

Alex North had perhaps dodged a bullet. Would Kubrick's film have triumphed with North's music? Would North's reputation have survived? Often, rejection is a sign that better things are on the horizon.

RECOMMENDED LISTENING

....

North – original soundtrack for *2001: A Space Odyssey*

⊙ *National Philharmonic Orchestra/Jerry Goldsmith (Varèse Sarabande)*

....

R

Resentment

Do you ever get that feeling that no matter how hard you try, no one will ever see things your way? During his lifetime, African-American composer Scott Joplin was one of the biggest names in music, his ragtime piano pieces such as *The Entertainer* (1902) and *Maple Leaf Rag* (1899) capturing the popular imagination for their brilliantly memorable tunes, addictive syncopations and sense of wry fun. Joplin wrote over 40 piano rags, all technically well within the grasp of decent amateur pianists. Classic miniatures such as *The Easy Winners* and *Elite Syncopations* made for perfect evening entertainment in the era before the gramophone, and the music sold in its hundreds of thousands, making Joplin a fortune. As jazz started to sweep across the United States, Joplin's music was viewed as the stepping stone from serious classical music to a freer, more decadent world.

The problem was, Joplin viewed himself as a serious classical composer and resented the way his rags were played too fast in order to highlight their jazziness. Yes, he enjoyed a blue note or two, but his rags were salon pieces to be played in a calm, relaxed manner. He would often write at the head of his scores, 'Note: Do not play this piece fast. It is never right to play "ragtime" fast. Composer.' Joplin even published a method book, *The School of Ragtime*, to try to persuade people to play his rags as written – but to no avail. Even today, Joplin's music is seen as a precursor to jazz, not helped by the likes of Jelly Roll Morton, who took rag out of the salon and into the night clubs, developing from it 'stride' piano.

In 1994, pianist Joshua Rifkin recorded a selection of Joplin's rags in the manner they were intended to be played. The results on his million-selling album are surprising – slow tempos, steady rhythms and an altogether gentle demeanour. Listening to Rifkin, and particularly his laid-back, stately approach

R

to *The Entertainer*, it is easy to understand how resentful Joplin must have felt to see his music wrongly labelled and pushed in a direction that diluted his ambitions to be a respected classical musical figure. If Joplin had been alive to hear these recordings, his resentment may well have subsided. And with a little empathy, Rifkin's performance of *The Entertainer* can help us all put our grudges in perspective.

RECOMMENDED LISTENING

Joplin – *The Entertainer*

⊙ *Joshua Rifkin (piano) (Nonesuch)*

Resilience (lack of)

The horrors of the 20th century have given composers many chances to portray the human spirit at its most resilient. Within the walls of Terezín, however, music went hand in hand with extraordinary displays of human courage and strength. Between 1941 and 1945, the Czech town was ghettoized by the Nazis and turned into a concentration camp. Among its 60,000 prisoners there thrived an extraordinary musical culture, which included performances by Alice Herz-Sommer, a Jewish pianist who died in 2014 at the astonishing age of 110. 'When I played,' she recalled, 'we felt we were nearer to God.' Within Terezín's walls, composers such as Pavel Haas, Gideon Klein and Viktor Ullmann produced thrilling music in the face of unspeakable terror, the latter writing song cycles, piano sonatas, string quartets, even an opera. Haas's resolute *Study for Strings* is typical of their fearless work. Haas and Ullmann died at Auschwitz, Klein at the Fürstengrube concentration camp.

French composer Olivier Messiaen's *Quartet for the End of Time* emerged from his time as a prisoner in 1940 at Stalag VIII-A, a prisoner of war camp on the German–Polish border. Messiaen later revealed that 'only music made me survive the cruelty and horrors of the camp.' It was thanks to a guard that Messiaen was able to access manuscript paper – after six months of work on a battered old upright piano, the composer completed his remarkable *Quartet*, scored for the resources he had at his disposal: piano, violin, clarinet and cello. Messiaen and three French musician friends performed it in front of 5,000 fellow prisoners. The *Quartet for the End of Time* is sublime – beautiful and intensely spiritual.

The final two movements are a breathtaking expression of the composer's unshakeable faith and determination. Be inspired by the iridescent shimmer of the 'Fouillis d'arcs-en-ciel, pour l'ange qui annonce la fin du temps' ('Cluster of rainbows, for the angel who announces the end of time'), which melts into the supplicatory final movement, 'Louange à l'éternité de Jésus' ('Praise to the immortality of Jesus').

RECOMMENDED LISTENING

....

Messiaen – Quartet for the End of Time

 Martin Fröst (clarinet), Lucas Debargue (piano), Janine Jansen (violin), Torleif Thedéen (cello) (Sony)

....

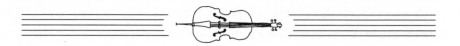

S

Sadness

If you are looking for a composer to join you in your sadness, you can do no better than to seek out the music of Shakespeare's contemporary John Dowland. Song titles such as 'Come, Heavy Sleep', 'Flow My Tears' and 'In Darkness Let Me Dwell' join the consort piece *Semper Dowland, Semper Dolens* ('Dowland, the ever-sorrowful'), giving the impression that the English composer was in an almost perpetual state of melancholy. Between 1597 and 1606, he may have had good reason to be. Failing to gain a position as a lutenist at the court of Elizabeth I (his friend the writer Henry Peacham later suggested that Dowland had 'slipt many opportunities in advancing his fortunes'), the composer found himself employed for nine years or so by King Christian IV of Denmark, a post that took him to Copenhagen without his wife and son.

Dowland wrote astounding chamber music exploring the complete range of human emotions, but there is no doubt that his pieces of a more downcast nature are on a genius plane. His music, often scored for voice and lute or lute alone, is full of sighing falls, descending harmonies and unexpected, exquisite harmonic twists that bring the listener's emotional pain to the surface. That is what makes Dowland's music the perfect companion for sadness – it is the 16th-century equivalent of a modern-day tearjerker.

Dowland's *Lachrimae Pavan* for five viols, later arranged by the composer himself for solo lute and as the song 'Flow My Tears', has been his most popular work since the 1580s. The Elizabethans considered melancholy to be one of the most fashionable of the 'humours', linked to introspection, thoughtfulness and genius (this was, after all, the age of Hamlet, Shakespeare's troubled prince), and Dowland's music seemed to embody all three qualities. The *Lachrimae Pavan*, the first piece in *Lachrimae*, Dowland's collection of pavans (processional dances) and other works, shares its opening descending four-note motif with much of the composer's melancholy music. Intended to evoke a slow-falling tear, Dowland's motif was copied by countless composers across Europe, determined to strike a similar gloomy chord. No one, however, could conjure such sublime sorrow as John Dowland.

RECOMMENDED LISTENING

Dowland – *Lachrimae Pavan*
◉ *Matthew Wadsworth (lute) (Channel Classics)*

Schadenfreude

While feeling cheerful at the idea of someone else's misery is not the most gallant of character traits, classical music can at least make you feel better about it. Opera, for instance, is full of such egregious characters that rejoicing at their downfall seems the only thing to do. There is something delicious about the misogynistic, abusive murderer Don Giovanni's final descent into hell at the end of Mozart's opera. And for a real feast of *Schadenfreude*, Richard Strauss's 1909 opera *Elektra* takes some beating. Everyone is ghastly, but Elektra's mother, the murderous adulterer Klytämnestra, and Elektra herself, hell-bent on a bloodthirsty revenge of her slain father, are portrayed with music of such grotesque savagery that it is more of a relief than a delight when both of them eventually meet their dramatic ends.

For *Schadenfreude* of a gentler nature, we are staying with Richard Strauss but moving away from opera to one of his greatest orchestral tone poems, *Till Eulenspiegel's Merry Pranks*. With orchestrations of sometimes mind-boggling invention, Strauss paints a vivid picture of Till Eulenspiegel, the 14th-century German folk hero – a sort of medieval vigilante who travels throughout Europe exposing corruption, vice, greed and so on, in the process humiliating an assortment of authority figures.

Strauss opens his tone poem with an ingenious musical 'once upon a time there was a buffoon', before a mischievous horn call announces Till's arrival. The whole piece is a succession of practical jokes on various people, including dour clergymen (represented by violas) and the 'cream of the philistines, the professors and savants' (heard in three growling bassoons, bass clarinet and contrabassoon). Justice eventually catches up with Till, who is caught and sentenced to die by hanging in some of Strauss's most thrillingly descriptive music. But even in death our hero has the final say, with the 'once upon a time' theme appearing once again before Till shoves two fingers up at the world.

In *Till Eulenspiegel*, Strauss was having a pop at the 'bankers and tradesmen of low tastes', as he put it, who had shown very little interest in his early work. His aim was to create for his audiences 'the most triumphant laughter in music' – and what could be funnier than sending up a few hypocritical solemn officials?

RECOMMENDED LISTENING

Strauss – *Till Eulenspiegel's Merry Pranks*
⊙ *Tonhalle Orchestra Zurich/David Zinman (Arte Nova)*

Secrecy

Post-Reformation, 16th-century England was not a safe place for Catholics, but many were determined to continue their traditions, despite the 1559 Act of Uniformity forbidding private Catholic worship. It was relatively easy to keep private prayer a secret, but things got a lot harder if you had your heart set on a full-scale Mass with music. With the help of elaborate priest holes and small chapels hidden within vast country manors – including Ingatestone, the seat of William Byrd's patron, Baron John Petre – wealthy Catholic families could subvert the law, but the risks were enormous, with government informers constantly scouring the land. Utter secrecy was the name of the game if you wanted to avoid a lengthy prison sentence, torture or even a gruesome death.

A proper Mass, however, needed music. Byrd was the greatest choral composer of his time, and his three Latin *Masses*, for three, four and five vocal parts, are miracles of the genre, concisely scored with elaborate counterpoint that nevertheless gives precedence to the beauty of the liturgy. It is hard to believe that such exquisite music was written with almost no prospect of public performance, but Byrd was a devout Catholic. As important as the music itself was its dissemination, and the *Masses* were published without details of date, composer or printer. Byrd, however, had friends in high places – as well as Petre, the Earl of Worcester and Baron John Lumley also risked their lives by financing and supporting Byrd's career.

If you want to do something and ensure it remains under wraps, then it pays to be like Byrd and create a false trail. In a move of genius, he and fellow composer Thomas Tallis schmoozed Queen Elizabeth I in 1575, securing a monopoly to print and publish music in any language. By way of thanks, the two of them produced the *Cantiones Sacrae*, a collection of 34 beautiful motets dedicated to the queen. With royal favour secured, how could Byrd possibly be suspected of illegal activity?

RECOMMENDED LISTENING

Byrd – *Masses for Three, Four and Five Voices*
⊙ *Westminster Cathedral Choir/Martin Baker (Hyperion)*

Selfishness

Sometimes it takes a person of standing to inspire us in acts of kindness. It is all very well knowing that our neighbours put out our trash bins while we are away, or shop regularly for the elderly couple across the road. But how much more powerful it is to learn that the actor George Clooney has been known to collect other people's parcels from the post office, or cancel their milk for them while they are away (even if he hasn't)?

Like George Clooney, Franz Liszt was once globally famous thanks to his extraordinary pianism and stage presence (see also page 95). Starting in 1841 in Berlin, 'Lisztomania', a term coined by the poet Heinrich Heine, was rife in Europe by 1842. Wherever he played, his recitals had more of the atmosphere of a pop concert than a civilized *soirée*, with adoring women in various states of hysteria fighting over the white gloves that Liszt threw into the crowd before he played. They even reportedly kept an eye on his half-drained glasses of water in the hope of drinking from the same cup as their musical god.

Underneath Liszt's theatrical veneer, however, was a man of great compassion and kindness. As early as 1832, one of his pupils, Madame Boissier, was describing his sense of social charity. 'He used to visit hospitals,' she wrote in

S

her diary, 'gambling dens and mental asylums, going down into the deepest dungeons and even talking to the men in the condemned cells.' Later in his career, Liszt gave away much of his recital income to various charities, and up until his retirement from the stage around 1865, he would often perform concerts to raise money for good causes.

But it was Liszt's support and nurturing of his fellow composers that went against the grain of the typically competitive artist. While Richard Wagner was in exile following the failed Dresden Uprising of 1849, for example, Liszt would conduct his opera overtures in concert in an attempt to keep his music in the public eye. And in 1877, Liszt brought to Weimar two composers he admired – Alexander Borodin and Camille Saint-Saëns. Of Saint-Saëns, Liszt said that he knew 'no one among contemporary artists who, taking everything into account, is his equal in talent, knowledge and diversity of skills', and it was in large part due to Liszt that Saint-Saëns's opera *Samson and Delila* made its Weimar debut by the end of the year.

For music both possessing a benign character and the power to inspire kindness, listen to the wonderful *Piano Concerto No. 1*, full of drama and passion and technical daring, but also some of the most charming moments in all Liszt's music.

RECOMMENDED LISTENING

Liszt – Piano Concerto No. 1

⊙ *Martha Argerich (piano), London Symphony Orchestra/Claudio Abbado*

Seriousness (excessive)

Classical music has a reputation for taking itself far too seriously. Much of the blame for that can probably be placed at the door of modern concert etiquette, which demands that hundreds of people sit in rows for a couple of hours, listening to performances in absolute silence and completely motionless. Latecomers will not be admitted. And if that quirky piece of Beethoven or Schubert should make you want to laugh out loud, restrain yourself. Enjoying a performance today is all about keeping a tight rein on your emotions, not just for the sake of your fellow concertgoers, but to avoid distracting the performers, most of whom have grown up unable to play in anything other than the most sterile conditions. For some, a jiggling leg in the front row is enough to put them off their stride. And God forbid you should clap in the wrong place, a concert convention that sent John F Kennedy into such a spin at White House concerts that he instructed his secretary to close a door in his sightline when it was time to applaud.

It never used to be like that. As recently as 1895, when the London Proms started as Mr Robert Newman's Promenade Concerts, audience members were free to mill around, eating and drinking (although they were requested not to strike matches during vocal performances). Franz Liszt's concerts were a riot of theatrical bravado and swooning ladies (see page 143). It is likely that neither Bach's congregations nor Haydn's employers sat listening in the same reverential, almost virtue-signalling way we do today. Somehow, in the past 100 years, classical music has been transformed from a popular art form into a club that excludes anyone who does not know and follow its arcane rules.

When violinist Nigel Kennedy released his EMI recording of Antonio Vivaldi's *The Four Seasons* back in 1989, it sent shockwaves throughout the classical music world. Here was a virtuoso with a cockney accent (shock, horror) and a spiky hairdo who refused to treat Vivaldi's four concertos like museum pieces, performing them in a way that made them feel more like street music than concert works. This was Vivaldi released from its shackles, performed by musicians who revelled in his vibrant depictions of the changing seasons with unbridled energy and joy. Surely that is how audiences should be able to show their appreciation of classical music.

RECOMMENDED LISTENING

Vivaldi – *The Four Seasons*
⊙ *Nigel Kennedy (violin), English Chamber Orchestra (Warner Classics)*

Sex (lack of)

We do not want to pry, but if you and your significant other have not been enjoying as much action between the sheets as you would both like, then perhaps it is time to do something about it. You may have given the tried and tested methods a shot – sexy lingerie, food of an aphrodisiacal nature, perhaps a temporary halt to all that bickering. But have you got the right music lined up? Setting the mood is crucial, and although Barry White, Marvin Gaye or the whisperings of Jane Birkin and Serge Gainsbourg might do it for some, we think something a little more subtle might prove more effective for the build-up.

Gone are the days, thank goodness, of choosing music long enough so as not to have to turn the record over, but compiling a digital playlist is also fraught with dangers. Although sudden changes in mood can put you back to square one, you don't want to bore each other either. Here is a feast of five pieces for guaranteed success.

Rodrigo – 'Adagio' from *Concierto de Aranjuez*

The guitar is surely the sexiest instrument of them all. The second movement of Joaquín Rodrigo's *Concerto* is sultry, passionate and ever so slightly agitated. We all like a bit of Spanish heat.

⊙ *Julian Bream (guitar), Monteverdi Orchestra/John Eliot Gardiner (Dutton)*

Debussy – *Prélude à l'après-midi d'un faune*

The French rival the Spanish for conjuring sexy moods. Claude Debussy's 12-minute, erotically charged orchestral work shimmers and glistens as our faun gets himself all worked up over a couple of nymphs, before sinking into a deep sleep.

⊙ *Sinfonia of London/John Wilson (Chandos)*

Scriabin – *The Poem of Ecstasy*

The Russians can play sexy, too, although Aleksandr Scriabin's 20-minute orchestral work is a little more frisky. It does, however, build up to two formidable climaxes, for want of a better word, which you will be lucky to improve upon.

⊙ *Philadelphia Orchestra/Riccardo Muti (Warner Classics)*

Chopin – *Prelude No. 15 'Raindrop'*

If all this orchestral intensity is putting you off more than turning you on, then try Frédéric Chopin's piano music, which is full of romance, just on a smaller scale. Listen to this *Prelude* for calm before and after the storm.

⊙ *Ingrid Fliter (piano) (Linn)*

Wagner – *Tristan and Isolde*

If you are aiming for a drought-busting, four-hour session, then pop on Richard Wagner's opera of love and lust, with its continuous crashing waves of desire –

although the ultimate climax comes in the rather unsexily named 'Liebestod' or 'love death' movement.

⊙ *Fritz Uhl and Birgit Nilsson, Vienna Philharmonic/Georg Solti (Decca)*

Sexism

When Ethel Smyth's brilliant four-movement *Violin Sonata* was first performed in 1887, it met with what today would be viewed as an outrageous response, with one critic suggesting that it was 'deficient in the feminine charm... expected of a woman composer'. Life was tough enough for any musician in Victorian England; for a female musician, the mountain to success was an almost impossible climb. Smyth, however, was undaunted, writing formidable works including her fine, Brahmsian *String Quintet* of 1883 and, decades later, a *String Quartet* that shows her at her mature best, and which owes much of its advanced style to Bartók. All the while, her no-nonsense approach and steely determination saw her cut a swathe through social norms, and by the turn of the 20th century, Smyth had become one of the most respected and recognizable composing names in the UK.

The more successful she became, the more she recognized her duty to stand up for her fellow women. She joined the Suffragette movement, for which she wrote the rousing *March of the Women*. Imprisoned in 1912 for throwing stones through the windows of a Member of Parliament, she spent two months in London's Holloway Prison. But even incarceration could not keep her down: from the window of her cell, according to the conductor Thomas Beecham, who was visiting her that day, Smyth could be seen conducting her fellow inmates with a toothbrush as they bellowed out her *March* in the exercise yard below.

For a taste of Smyth's extraordinary music, listen to her *Mass in D*, a work the composer once performed to Queen Victoria in a private concert that involved Smyth playing the piano while singing as many vocal parts as she could. In its intended form, for chorus and orchestra, the *Mass* fizzes with colour, its dazzling 'Gloria' a symbol of a composer who challenged the system and won.

RECOMMENDED LISTENING

Smyth – *Mass in D*
◉ *BBC Symphony Orchestra and Chorus/Sakari Oramo (Chandos)*

Sloth

If you have not done a great deal of exercise in recent years and plan on changing all that, you are going to want to take things slowly and increase your activity step by step. Start with a little stretching, a few brisk walks, gradually working up to a slow jog. Before you know it, you will be sprinting a 5km run and planning your first marathon. The music that is pumped into our gyms, however, does not encourage the gentle approach, as its fast, relentless beat hammers out the same punishing pulse from start to finish.

For those who feel a little slothlike, you might want to consider the following pieces, all of which start out at a snail's pace before finishing in a burst like Usain Bolt. Perfect for the reformed sloth.

Grieg – *In the Hall of the Mountain King*
Part of Edvard Grieg's incidental music to Ibsen's play *Peer Gynt*, 'In the Hall of the Mountain King' begins tentatively in the lower registers of the orchestra

before accelerating to a frantic, *fortissimo* finish. At just three minutes, it is an efficient way to get you off the sofa.

⊙ *Estonian National Symphony Orchestra/Paavo Järvi (Warner Classics)*

Rossini – 'Overture' from *William Tell*

A mournful solo cello sings out a lonely melody. Then before you know it, Giaochino Rossini is whipping up a storm with bombastic brass and woodwind. Calm is soon restored, but the high energy then returns in the form of one of the most famous gallops in all music.

⊙ *Orchestra dell'Accademia Nazionale di Santa Cecilia/Antonio Pappano (Warner Classics)*

Liszt – *Hungarian Rhapsody No. 2*

A melancholic, folk song-inspired introduction spans the first five minutes of Franz Liszt's *Hungarian Rhapsody No. 2*, after which a *friska*, a fast Hungarian dance, sends the music into a relentless spin that is impossible to resist.

⊙ *Budapest Festival Orchestra/Iván Fischer (Philips)*

Ravel – *La Valse*

The murmurings that start Maurice Ravel's biting satire of pre-First World War decadence begin one of classical music's most magnificent series of *crescendos*. They finally end, like all of us after exercise, exhausted in a crumpled heap.

⊙ *Rotterdam Philharmonic Orchestra/Yannick Nézet-Séguin (Warner Classics)*

S

Bach – 'Allegro' from *Brandenburg Concerto No. 3*

Presumably now all signs of slothfulness are well and truly banished. To keep up your momentum, listen to Johann Sebastian Bach's first movement – something with oodles of energy and, crucially, metronomically constant from the start, like a musical chugging engine.

⊙ *European Brandenburg Ensemble/Trevor Pinnock (Avie)*

Stamina (lack of)

Why are we able to binge dozens of hours of series box sets or devour 1,000-page novels, yet find the idea of sitting through Mahler's Third Symphony less than appealing? For some reason, listening, rather than reading or watching, demands more from us. That is why it is easier to enjoy a Bruckner symphony while travelling, whether walking, running, driving or taking the train, than while sitting quietly – travel gives our eyes something to do while our ears are occupied. And it is one of the reasons conductors are so important – in the concert hall, they provide a focal point, a visual diversion in the music's less than thrilling moments. Nevertheless, to listen to a symphony from start to finish while doing nothing else is to engage with it in its purest way. And without visual distractions, you will almost certainly notice more detail in the score.

A symphony or string quartet does not present the ultimate endurance test – there are far greater challenges. Anyone who has emerged unfrazzled from a performance of Erik Satie's *Vexations*, either in their home or on the rare instances when it has been performed in a concert hall, should pat themselves on the back. Written in the 1890s, *Vexations* consists of a short piece of chromatic piano music played 840 times, with an authentic performance lasting around 28 hours.

This is nothing compared to John Cage's *Organ²/ASLSP (As Slow as Possible)*, currently being performed on a primitive pipe organ in the church of St Burchardi in Halberstadt, Germany. Cage gives no clue to how slow the piece should actually be played, which means that performances can last from mere minutes to, in this case, hundreds of years. Curtain down at St Burchardi is set for the year 2640, with small chord changes happening almost every year as pipes are added or removed from the wind chest. It has not yet been decided whether there will be an interval.

S

RECOMMENDED LISTENING

Satie – *Vexations*

⊙ *Jeroen van Veen (piano) (Brilliant Classics)*

Stinginess

Music has the power to improve your mood. A quick burst of sunny Corelli, some breezy Haydn, perhaps some gentle Vaughan Williams has almost limitless powers to cheer us up. If music can make us happy, and happiness makes us more empathetic and therefore predisposed to larger restaurant tips, giving to charity and all-round good deeds, can music directly make us more generous? As it happens, it probably can. Various pieces of scientific research have already pointed to music making us socially more generous: lowering levels of classroom noise, assuaging individuals' aggression towards others and just generally making us more likely to help our fellow humans.

In 2014, two Japanese professors of education, Hajime Fukui and Kumiko Toyoshima, selected 11 men and 11 women to play the Dictator Game, an apparently simple psychological test whereby a 'dictator' decides how much money to give to a passive recipient. The game was played while a variety of relaxing musical pieces were played, chosen either by the dictator or the recipient. The results were fascinating, with dictators giving more money away when listening to their favourite 'chilled' music, especially when they believed the track had been chosen by the recipient. They gave less money away when played music they actively disliked.

We should all be more generous, so here are five chill-inducing works to help you dig into those pockets a little bit deeper.

Beethoven – 'Adagio un poco mosso' from *Piano Concerto No. 5* ('*Emperor*')

A hushed orchestral introduction gives way to one of Ludwig van Beethoven's most mesmerizing works as the piano enters, starting from on high before meandering downwards, beautifully aimless.

⊙ *Alfred Brendel (piano), Vienna Philharmonic Orchestra/Simon Rattle (Decca)*

Delius – *On Hearing the First Cuckoo in Spring*

The English composer Frederick Delius's meltingly gorgeous tone poem is a pastoral masterpiece, the subtle, exotic string harmonies framing the cuckoo, which peeks through the textures as if heard from across a valley.

⊙ *Hallé Orchestra/Mark Elder (Hallé)*

Fauré – 'Prelude' from *Pelléas et Mélisande*

Gabriel Fauré's orchestral suite is full of wonderful tunes, including the ravishing 'Sicilienne', but it is the prelude that rises like the sun on a misty spring day.

⊙ *Academy of St Martin in the Fields/Neville Marriner (Decca)*

Whitacre – *Lux Aurumque*

The American choral composer Eric Whitacre writes choral music of ravishing beauty, with harmonic suspensions galore and wide, generous chords that create a wall of hypnotic sound. *Lux Aurumque* is one of his finest.

⊙ *Eric Whitacre Singers (Decca)*

S

Massenet – 'Méditation' from *Thaïs*

Jules Massenet's exquisite interlude for violin and orchestra is played in Act II of the opera as the beautiful Thaïs ponders the monk Athanaël's invitation to forsake her life of luxury for God.

⊙ *Renaud Capuçon (violin) (Erato)*

Stress

For the generation whose parents grew up with cheap housing, free education, jobs for life and generous pensions, life may be very stressful. Even when we have got on to the first rung of the property ladder, we still need to pay the mortgage, and those with children are caught in an extra spiral of cleaning, cooking and discipline. If you miraculously find time to sit down with a glass or two of wine of an evening, here are some works to help you forget the impossibilities of modern living and reduce those stress levels, if only for an hour or so.

Delius – *The Walk to the Paradise Garden*
An extract from Frederick Delius's rarely performed opera *A Village Romeo and Juliet*, this beautiful, soft-hued orchestral interlude describes a stroll not to a beautiful garden, but to a pub. And what could be more stress-relieving that a slow meander towards a pint of amber ale?
⊙ *Royal Liverpool Philharmonic Orchestra/John Wilson (Avie)*

Grainger – *Blithe Bells*
Percy Grainger transforms Johann Sebastian Bach's aria 'Sheep May Safely Graze', from his secular cantata *Was Mir Behagt*, into a beautiful, grandly scored orchestral ramble. There are exotic, delicious harmonies, the gentle plink of the celeste, lush strings – what more could you want? Feel that stress melt away.
⊙ *BBC Philharmonic/Richard Hickox (Chandos)*

Granados – 'Quejas ó la maja y el ruiseñor' from *Goyescas*
Music that takes away stress need not be devoid of passion. 'The Maiden and the Nightingale', a beautiful movement from Enrique Granados's Goya-inspired

piano suite, has a yearning quality that never spills over into melodrama. Six minutes of dreaminess.

◉ *Nelson Freire (piano) (Decca)*

Bach – 'Chaconne' from *Partita No. 2 for Solo Violin*

Johann Sebastian Bach's 'Chaconne' is a musical miracle – an endlessly inventive, mesmerizing set of variations on a simple bass ground. Despite being scored for just one solo instrument, it is among the most emotional works ever written, and each listen will reveal something new.

◉ *Julia Fischer (violin) (Pentatone)*

Lauridsen – *O Magnum Mysterium*

Written for Christmastide, American composer Morten Lauridsen's slow-moving work for double choir is full of delicious suspensions and wide, earthy chords. If you are after some stress-relieving calmness, here it is.

◉ *Polyphony/Stephen Layton (Hyperion)*

S

T

Temptation

Temptation lurks around every corner in classical music. Composers including Liszt, Berlioz and Gounod in the 19th century had a field day with Goethe's *Faust*, their music the perfect conduit for its lurid tale of entrapment and seduction. Nothing, however, quite matches the astringent power of Igor Stravinsky's 1917 theatrical work, *The Soldier's Tale* – a remarkable, forthright piece of theatre that tells the story of a young soldier's downfall: one moment enjoying ten days' leave from the front, the next trading in his beloved fiddle for the promise of untold riches. It is a game of cat and mouse, as both soldier and Devil struggle throughout for the upper hand.

Stravinsky and a friend, the writer Charles Ferdinand Ramuz, conceived *The Soldier's Tale* as a quick way to make money. Both were stranded in Switzerland during the First World War, separated from international stages and music publishers, and this simple production of theirs could easily be taken around the country and performed from the back of a wagon. Its simplicity is its secret weapon. Ramuz's libretto, originally in French and divided between three actors (alongside a silent female dancer), tells its story in verse of remarkable triviality: 'Along a hot and dusty road / Tramps a soldier with his load. / Ten days' leave he has to spend. / Will his journey never end?' Then Stravinsky complements Ramuz's words with equally acerbic music performed by a pared-down ensemble of solo violin, wind instruments, brass and percussion. Martial rhythms mix with tango, ragtime with Russian folk songs, all at the mercy of Stravinsky's constantly shifting time signatures.

Like a circus clown, *The Soldier's Tale* is both comic and sinister, charming one moment, suffocating the next. In true Faustian style, there is no room for redemption, either. The soldier's final bid for freedom is met with the swaggering 'Triumphal March of the Devil'. Temptation has never come at so high a price.

RECOMMENDED LISTENING

Stravinsky – *The Soldier's Tale*
⊙ *John Gielgud (narrator), Tom Courtenay (The Soldier), Ron Moody (The Devil), Boston Symphony Chamber Players (Eloquence)*

Trust (lack of)

For thousands of years, people have played instruments and sung music together around a campfire – and for very good reason. Music engenders trust – it is a way to dispel suspicions and create a social glue. It is almost as if the guitarist or drummer is testing us: sing along, and you are one of us; stay silent, and we will tread carefully around you. Music is important to a balanced, trusting society, and the science backs it up. A key to generating trust, according to scientists at the University of Oxford, is to synchronize our musical experiences with those of others. Doing so creates a common goal, which in turn prompts our brain to generate endorphins, the chemicals that produce feelings of pleasure in the brain.

T

Throughout history, music has been a social activity centred around a shared rhythm, from centuries-old dance forms to a stadium crowd clapping along to a hit song. It is why ensembles simply must trust one another – you cannot make great music with unreliable or disliked colleagues. Witness how often some string quartets change their personnel.

Increasingly, music is being used by companies to improve levels of trust within the workplace. Particularly effective are singing courses, whereby participants not only overcome their nervousness of singing in public, but also learn to sing in basic harmony by listening to and relying on each other. Rounds are a great way to form a bond with others, even pieces as simple as 'Frère Jacques' or 'London's Burning'. Rhythm-based pieces, however, whether drummed or clapped, are even better – people are far more ready to clap or bash something in public than they are to sing.

For some inspiration, listen to minimalist composer Steve Reich's three-minute *Clapping Music*, a thrilling one-movement work that requires total cooperation and complete trust between the two performers. The piece consists of a basic rhythm clapped by one of the performers for the duration of the piece. The other performer starts with the same pattern, but every 8 or 12 bars they shift by a quaver (an eighth note), moving further and further out of sync with their partner to create complex polyrhythms. A successful performance relies on a lot of practice – and a good deal of trust.

RECOMMENDED LISTENING

Reich – *Clapping Music*
◉ *Colin Currie, Steve Reich (Colin Currie Records)*

U

Unruliness

We could all do with a spot of unruliness in our lives – not necessarily to have the most fun, but for the chaos that happens around it. The same is true in classical music, although there used to be many more opportunities for musicians to run amok than there are now. Back in 18th-century Germany, for instance, organists would regularly improvise voluntaries (pieces of church music), making daring use of huge, multi-manual instruments and prodigious finger and pedal techniques. And in Mozart's day, improvising concerto cadenzas was seen as a necessary part of the job. Today, things are a little more prescriptive, and even star performers have their moments of glory written out for them in full.

Thankfully, there are still pockets of disorderliness lurking in the repertoire. Percussionists have Danish composer Carl Nielsen to thank for one of classical music's most powerful anarchic moments. Nielsen's *Symphony No. 5* was written in the years following the First World War. The war itself had been a strange one for Denmark – it had stayed neutral throughout but was no doubt nervous about the threat from the country on its southern border. As Nielsen watched the war unfold from afar, so his faith in the idea of nationalism was sorely shaken. It had, he lamented, resulted in 'senseless hate'.

The first movement is a mighty struggle between good and evil, its opening minutes almost Vaughan Williams-esque in style – no hint of angst here. Soon the clouds gather, however, the mood darkening bar by bar into a sparseness more reminiscent of Shostakovich, before the idyll is shattered by the martial beats of a side drum – and then calm descends. But before long the side drum returns, its disruptive power greatly magnified as the player is encouraged by Nielsen to improvise 'in his own tempo, as though determined at all costs to obstruct the music'. It is a fierce, uncompromising moment, all the more shocking for the sheer contrast of this unfettered, violent outburst set against the chorale-like textures of the underlying orchestra, fighting to be heard above the free-for-all.

RECOMMENDED LISTENING

Nielsen – *Symphony No. 5*
⊙ *London Symphony Orchestra/Colin Davis (LSO Live)*

Urban malaise

For those of us who live and work in the city, life can be noisy and relentless, and at some point we have all yearned to escape to the country. One thing we dream of is the sound of birdsong, unaffected by traffic noise, joyful in its celebration of fresh air and surfeit of space. Limited to the 12 tones of Western notation, many composers have incorporated an approximation of birdsong into their music – most notably the 20th-century Frenchman Olivier Messiaen, whose *Catalogue d'Oiseaux* sketches the songs of 77 birds native to France with piano writing of astonishing descriptive power and harmonic invention. The musical language is often dissonant, the pieces themselves a little tricky to access, but persevere and you will realize what a master craftsman is Messiaen – who proves that despite its limitations, music can bring the grasshopper warbler, golden oriole, blue rock thrush and many more birds to mesmerizing life.

For a real sense of wild, untamed nature, however, seek out Einojuhani Rautavaara's 1972 work, *Cantus Arcticus*. The Finnish composer lays a foundation of orchestral sound over which he places a pre-recorded track of a variety of Arctic birds, avoiding the problem of recreating their sound for instruments. Divided into three movements – 'The Bog', 'Melancholy' and 'Swans Migrating' – *Cantus Arcticus* blends the sound of shore larks and other seabirds with vast orchestral landscapes that evoke desolate Finnish tundra and the biting wind that sweeps through the boreal forest and across the frozen lakes.

Head straight to 'Swans Migrating', which features a five-minute orchestral *crescendo* to the accompaniment of a chorus of whooper swans. Rautavaara overlaps blocks of sound in such a way that the music mimics the swans' V-shaped flight formation, each bird taking its turn at the front of the group. In the movement's dying minutes, the swans disappear over the horizon, Rautavaara's music following as it fades to silence, leaving in its wake the vast, silent wilderness of arctic Finland.

RECOMMENDED LISTENING

Rautavaara – *Cantus Arcticus*
⊙ *Royal Scottish National Orchestra/Hannu Lintu (Naxos)*

U

Uselessness (feelings of)

Accountants, lawyers, doctors, writers, any sort of manager – all of these jobs demand obvious and acknowledged skills. Pity, then, the poor players of, say, the contrabassoon, bass trombone or even the theremin. Their skills do not often see the light of day, much like those experts who are called upon by television news programmes every ten years to comment on a story about a rare bird or some niche corner of astrophysics. The art of banishing your feelings of utter uselessness lies in making the most of those rare times when you do get to bathe in the limelight. There are some wonderful concertos written for instruments that rarely get the chance to shine, which give their performers (and, by proxy, their listeners) a warm feeling of inclusivity and self-worth.

In 2005, Finnish composer Kalevi Aho took pity on said contrabassoonists with an eerie, Shostakovich-inspired epic, the *Contrabassoon Concerto*, that put the orchestra's deepest instruments in a whole new light. Unfortunately, he also put them on a whole new level, writing well beyond the contrabassoon's range. Luckily, the work's dedicatee, Lewis Lipnick, found a solution and subsequently declared Aho's work a triumph, helping the contrabassoon to 'sing as well as rumble'.

But the prize for uselessness surely goes to the early synthesizer, the Trautonium, of which Oskar Sala was the only champion, and perhaps the only player. Invented around 1929 by Friedrich Trautwein, the Trautonium's sound was produced by pressing keys that in turn touched a resistive wire at various point along its length. The sound it produced was a blend of saxophone and flugelhorn. It never took off, as it was not long before technology was coming up with better, more versatile electronic instruments. Paul Hindemith, however, was a fan, writing a set of seven short pieces for three Trautoniums and, in

1931, a full-blown *Concertino for Trautonium and String Orchestra*. That is, sadly, where the Trautonium's repertoire began and ended. But the piece itself is an unexpected neo-classical delight, making the most of the instrument's haunting tone, expressive potential and ability to sustain long lines. If it were not written for such an esoteric instrument, Hindemith's work would surely have gained wider currency.

RECOMMENDED LISTENING

Hindemith – *Concertino for Trautonium and String Orchestra*
⊙ *Oskar Sala (Trautonium), Munich Chamber Orchestra/Hans Stadlmair (Apex)*

U

Vanity

Music is composed to be heard. And a lot of music is intentionally written not just to be heard by thousands, but to be cheered by them, too. There is nothing a composer likes more than standing up at the end of a premiere, making their way to the stage and basking in the applause. Surely Gustav Mahler's *Symphony No. 8*, his 'Symphony of a Thousand', was not written simply to demonstrate the magnificence of its scoring and the ambitions of its musical and religious ideas. When he conducted 1,029 musicians at its 1910 premiere, was Mahler creating a huge arena for his ego? This was the same man who forbade his own wife, Alma, to compose, suggesting that her artistic ambitions were nothing but vanity. Mahler wanted all the attention for himself.

Away from such grand public statements, chamber music thrives in a more modest world, where audiences and ensembles are smaller and the music is sometimes performed for no one but the players themselves. There is one work, however, that was never intended to be played in any sort of concert hall or public place but is nevertheless regarded as one of its composer's finest works.

Camille Saint-Saëns was one of the greatest musicians of his age. He made his public debut at the age of ten performing a Mozart piano concerto, and offered to perform as an encore any Beethoven piano sonata – from memory. Years later, none other than the legendary pianist Franz Liszt hailed him as the best organist in the world. As a composer, Saint-Saëns was regarded as the 'French Beethoven', and yet much of his music, including piano concertos, symphonies and chamber music, is devoid of loftiness. There is no philosophical grandeur here – just good, solid music, brilliantly crafted.

As an ultimate show of modesty, Saint-Saëns wrote *The Carnival of the Animals* for a select group of colleagues and friends, who first performed it in private. In fact, the composer forbade the piece – scored for two pianos, two violins, viola, cello, double bass, flute, piccolo, clarinet, glass harmonica and xylophone – from being performed in public until after his death, fearing it might prove too popular. ('The Swan' was given special dispensation). All of Saint-Saëns's inventive wit is in the 14-movement suite, each instrument given its moment in the limelight, from the scampering pianos of 'Wild Donkeys' to the galumphing double bass in 'The Elephant'. The tinkling xylophone gets the cleverest movement, which features quotes from old nursery rhymes and operatic arias that the composer considered to be musical fossils.

It was only in 1922, a year after Saint-Saëns's death, that the French publisher Durand issued the work, in accordance with the composer's wishes; its first public performance was given in the same year. To this day, *The Carnival of the Animals* remains Saint-Saëns's most popular work – but one from which he declined to benefit.

RECOMMENDED LISTENING

Saint-Saëns – *The Carnival of the Animals*

⊙ *The Kanneh-Masons, with Michael Morpurgo and Olivia Colman (Decca)*

V

Vigour (lack of)

If you have ever been to a German health spa, you will know how fond Europeans are of the plunge pool. After the extreme heat of a dry sauna, a quick dip in some icy cold water releases endorphins, pumps the blood around the body and gets you ready for the day, invigorated. There is no reason why that cannot work with music, too.

First, some warmth. In 'Summer', from his set of four violin concertos, *The Four Seasons*, Antonio Vivaldi brings the season's stifling heat to feverish life, opening with wafts of hot air followed by strange, manic birdsong as 'Man and his flock languish, and the pine tree burns'. A swarm of insects makes an unwelcome entrance in the 'Adagio' before the final movement's gathering storm rips through the Mediterranean humidity (see also page 145). Vivaldi's music is extraordinary in its dramatic scope, as is the music of early 20th-century Spanish composer Manuel de Falla, whose impressionistic *Nights in the Gardens of Spain* takes us to Córdoba and Granada with music of sweeping, shimmering beauty, its hints of folk song and rippling solo piano adding to the hazy, dusky atmosphere.

By now you will be aching to cool off and dive into one of the 17th-century English composer Henry Purcell's supreme musical achievements: the Frost Scene from the opera *King Arthur*, a brilliant musical description of frosty winter. 'What Power Art Thou Who From Below', to give the aria its proper title, features stammering writing for bass solo and a spiky, shivering orchestral accompaniment as the Cold Genius is awakened in the dead of a bone-chilling English winter.

But if January on the North Sea coast still feels a little balmy, perhaps the Antarctic might do the trick. Ralph Vaughan Williams based his 1951 *Symphony*

No. 7 on the music he had written for the 1948 film *Scott of the Antarctic*. The music of 'Sinfonia Antartica', as it was named, is among the English composer's most dramatic, with wind machine and wordless voices in the first movement bringing the Antarctic's frozen, barren wastes to life. The third movement, 'Landscape', features towering glaciers courtesy of Vaughan Williams's iridescent orchestration, highlighting percussion, woodwind and brass, with the might of a pipe organ adding a colossal sense of scale and polar otherworldliness towards the end.

RECOMMENDED LISTENING

Vivaldi – 'Summer' from *The Four Seasons*

⊙ *Nigel Kennedy (violin), English Chamber Orchestra (Warner Classics)*

De Falla – *Nights in the Gardens of Spain*

⊙ *Steven Osborne (piano), BBC Scottish Symphony Orchestra/Ludovic Morlot*

Purcell – 'Frost Scene' from *King Arthur*

⊙ *Gabrieli Players/Paul McCreesh (Signum)*

Vaughan Williams – *Symphony No. 7 'Sinfonia Antartica'*

⊙ *BBC Symphony Orchestra/Andrew Davis (Warner Classics)*

V

Vulnerability

We all have our weak spots – situations or things that can pierce our armour and remind us that we are human. It is the reason many of us stick to what we are good at: the still life painter who steers away from portraiture, the writer who never attempts fiction, the chef who avoids soufflés like the plague. The same is true for musicians: only the brave attempt everything in their instrument's repertoire. Indeed, one of the finest pianists ever to have lived, Murray Perahia, has never recorded any of the Rachmaninov piano concertos. Nor has the renowned Baroque violinist Rachel Podger played the Tchaikovsky *Violin Concerto* in public. It may be because she does not want to, but it could equally be because Tchaikovsky demands things of her technique that she has not developed. Each to their own.

There is, however, one composer from whom no musician can escape, no matter what their instrument or specialism. Such is the timelessness of 18th-century composer Johann Sebastian Bach's music that he is rarely referred to as a 'Baroque' composer. He is simply a composer, one who speaks to all ages, which is why all musicians feel compelled to play his music. Nevertheless, even the best technicians will admit that Bach is very hard to play, his contrapuntal complexities and transparent textures requiring utter precision. To the listener, Bach's music sounds effortless; to the player, much of it is like climbing a rock face with the smallest of footholds. One slip and the whole performance can come tumbling down. For cellists and violinists, who normally play in ensembles or with pianists, the works for solo cello and solo violin can instil fear.

It is no wonder so many musicians only turn to certain Bach works late in their careers. After all, Bach can define a musician like no other composer. Cellist Steven Isserlis, acclaimed in so much repertoire from Brahms to Shostakovich,

V

only recorded the *Cello Suites* at the age of 48, while pianist Daniel Barenboim waited until he was 64 before releasing his first recording of Books 1 and 2 of *The Well-Tempered Clavier*. Even the very best of us need time to face up to our vulnerabilities.

RECOMMENDED LISTENING

Bach – *Six Cello Suites*

⊙ *Steven Isserlis (cello) (Hyperion)*

V

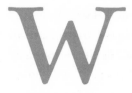

Waking up (difficulty in)

Late nights, long work hours or a new baby are just a few of the many reasons why you might be feeling a little jaded this morning. Alarm clocks are getting cleverer at waking us up more gently – now it is only the masochistic among us who rise to the deafening sound of a mechanical alarm or the hellish shriek of a digital clock radio. Nevertheless, there are better ways to wake up feeling fresh and bright-eyed, and music is one of them. The right piece can be the aural equivalent of those bedside lamps that simulate the gradually brightening light of the rising sun.

Scene III of Maurice Ravel's deeply sensuous 1912 ballet, *Daphnis et Chloé*, begins with one of the most magical sunrises in all of music. In 'Lever du jour' ('Daybreak'), Ravel captures the sound of morning dew trickling over rocks with exquisite skill, flutes cascading above a pastel wash of shifting, languorous strings. The slowly rising sun catches on the water, while awakening birds sing to a new day from the trees. Daphnis, catching sight of Chloé, rushes into her arms. The sun rises, gloriously but not too dramatically, accompanied by an ethereal wordless chorus. You will want to stay in bed and listen to the whole scene, but you have work to do.

If you prefer waking to something a little more wintry and rugged, then the opening of Richard Strauss's *An Alpine Symphony* is equally vivid. This epic

1915 tone poem takes the listener on an 11-hour ascent and stormy descent of a mountain, setting off before sunrise. Rumbling brass, strings and low woodwind evoke the looming presence of the mountain in darkness, note clusters and snatches of brass fanfares rising slowly in both pitch and volume, before a glorious theme pierces the gloom as the morning sun glistens on the snowy peaks. Strauss's music continues busily through foothills, woods and past a waterfall for some minutes – so there is no chance of you falling asleep again.

We turn, finally, to the English seaside town of Eastbourne and to Ravel's fellow Impressionist, Claude Debussy, who wrote much of his orchestral suite *La Mer* while on holiday in 1904, enjoying the company of a lady who most definitely was not his wife. Debussy's progression in the opening movement from dawn to midday features a longer *crescendo* than Strauss employs at the start of his *Alpine Symphony*, but you certainly know when the sun reaches its zenith. In the minutes before, you can almost smell the swelling, churning sea, the wind whipping up whitecaps, the light refracted through the spray. It is a stunning evocation of nature that preludes a morning shower rather nicely.

Ravel – *Daphnis et Chloé*
⊙ *Orchestre et Choeur de l'Opéra National de Paris/Philippe Jordan (Erato)*

....

Strauss – *An Alpine Symphony*
⊙ *Concertgebouw Orchestra/Bernard Haitink (Philips)*

....

Debussy – *La Mer*
⊙ *The Cleveland Orchestra/Pierre Boulez (Deutsche Grammophon)*

....

W

Weepiness

There is nothing like a good cry, and in times of sadness we do not always want cheering up. It is often far better to watch a good old classic film and bawl our eyes out. The same is true for classical music, which has an almost bottomless supply of weepies.

Like film, music affects different people in different ways. Some of us might be triggered by the sheer quality of the piece, in a reaction known as Stendhal Syndrome; we may find our chosen music so beautiful as to be emotionally overwhelming. Alternatively, it may be the underlying sentiment in it that affects us, or even an unusual harmony that sets us off. Or, as with the final emphatic chorus in Bach's *St Matthew Passion* or the appearance of the placid 'Nimrod' in Elgar's otherwise bustling *Enigma Variations* (see page 103), a release of musical tension helps us reach for the hankies.

We cannot second-guess the music to make you cry, but here are five pieces that will almost surely make you reach for a tissue. Go on – let it all out. You'll feel much better.

Brahms – *Intermezzo in C Sharp Minor*
Much of Johannes Brahms's piano makes the cut, including most of the *Intermezzos* – works of deep introspection and loneliness.
◉ *Radu Lupu (piano) (Decca)*

Vaughan Williams – *Fantasia on a Theme of Thomas Tallis*
A gorgeously over-orchestrated fantasy by Ralph Vaughan Williams on an ancient tune. Its sheer sumptuousness is enough to bring you to tears.
◉ *BBC Symphony Orchestra/Andrew Davis (Warner Classics)*

Beethoven – 'Andante cantabile' from *Piano Sonata No. 8 'Pathétique'*
One of Ludwig van Beethoven's most beautiful themes is accompanied by rich, deep harmonies that never fail to satisfy. Perhaps its scoring in the key of A flat is a clue to its poignancy.

⊙ *Igor Levit (piano) (Sony Classical)*

....

Prokofiev – 'Romeo and Juliet's Love Dance' from *Romeo and Juliet*
No one has captured the sheer beauty of the passion between Shakespeare's star-cross'd lovers as deeply and movingly as Sergei Prokofiev. This movement is particularly weepy.

⊙ *London Symphony Orchestra/Valery Gergiev (LSO Live)*

....

Elgar – *Cello Concerto*
As Edward Elgar hummed the opening, whispered theme on his deathbed, he said to his friend W H Reed, 'If you're ever walking on the Malvern Hills and hear it, don't be frightened – it's only me.'

⊙ *Paul Watkins (cello), BBC Philharmonic/Andrew Davis*

....

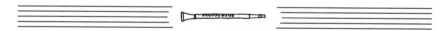

W

Wit (excessive use of)

Is there such a thing as too much wit? Not necessarily, but if you are going to be funny all the time, you need a constant source of original material and a knack of knowing your audience. It helps to be liked, too. No one achieved all these things – and more – better than the 18th-century composer Joseph Haydn.

Haydn was a one-man music revolutionary, single-handedly inventing and perfecting the string quartet genre, while his 104 symphonies contain so many sparkling ideas that their influence stretched far into the 19th century. And in so much of his music, Haydn pursued a sense of fun – from moments of slapstick to subtle, knowing allusions, the Austrian was a natural, with a huge comedic range, for whom wit and musical perfection went hand in hand.

You can hear gentle teasing at play, for instance, in the Op. 33 *String Quartets*, with No. 2's false endings that brilliantly wrong-foot the listener, or the grace notes that give No. 3 a whimsical, chirruping character.

But it is in his symphonies that Haydn displays his full comic potential, including the industrial-action-in-music 'Farewell' Symphony (*Symphony No. 45*), at the end of which the musicians leave the stage one by one, originally in protest at their working conditions. Their employer, Prince Esterházy, took the joke in good grace. Then there is the 'Surprise' Symphony (*Symphony No. 94*), whose sudden thwack on the timpani halfway through its 'Andante' second movement gives dozing audience members a heart-pounding jolt. Elsewhere, Haydn raises a smile and a chuckle simply on account of his originality and daring: an unexpected drum roll at the start of *Symphony No. 103* or, in *Symphony No. 80*, a culture clash of *Sturm und Drang* brooding intensity and a simple courtly dance. As ever, Haydn takes wit to a new level.

W

RECOMMENDED LISTENING

Haydn – String Quartets Op. 33

⊙ *Quatuor Mosaïques (Naïve)*

Workaholism

There are prolific composers, and then there is Johann Sebastian Bach. When the German Baroque composer was appointed music director of St Thomas's Church in Leipzig in 1723, he may have felt compelled to prove his worth after learning he was fourth choice for the role and that the favourite, the celebrated Georg Telemann, had turned it down. Just weeks after setting foot in the city, Bach became a composing machine: for the first two years at Leipzig he turned out at least one full-scale, multi-movement church cantata every Sunday, usually scored for orchestra, organ, choir and vocal soloists – more than 90 works, each a mini-opera. It was a massive undertaking, a self-imposed workload that produced reams of music of incredible originality, each note fitting its liturgical purpose like a glove. Yet writing them was just the start. Dozens of music parts had to be copied out for the singers and orchestral musicians, and everything had to be thoroughly rehearsed.

As if that was not enough, over the years Bach put time aside to write some of Western music's greatest masterworks, including three *Passions* – the *St Matthew*, the *St John* and the now lost *St Mark* – as well as the glorious *Mass in B Minor* (see page 52), the *Magnificat* and major pieces for the pipe organ. How did Bach explain his creative fertility? 'I worked hard,' he said with infuriating modesty towards the end of his life. 'Anyone who works as hard as I did can achieve the same results.'

W

Bach maintained his momentum for years, using family and friends for menial copying tasks and senior choristers for rehearsal duties. The simple truth, however, is that he could not keep it up, and there are signs that he started to take short cuts. Paying a friend to teach his Latin lessons was just the beginning – it gradually dawned on him that digging out existing cantatas and repurposing them for different liturgical occasions would more than fulfil expectations. The clergy and congregation, perhaps even the musicians, would not even notice.

And so it was that in 1734 Bach turned his attention to a series of cantatas to run from Christmas Day to Epiphany – the *Christmas Oratorio*, one of the festive season's most joyous works exploring Christmastide's major feast days. The first few bars of the opening chorus 'Jauchzet, frohlocket' are a thrilling union of cascading strings, brass fanfares and thundering drum. But for all its richness and invention, the *Christmas Oratorio* is, in fact, plundered from several previously composed secular cantatas, including 213, 214 and 215 in the catalogue of Bach's works. Even music's workaholics know when to work smarter rather than harder (see also page 69).

RECOMMENDED LISTENING

Bach – *Christmas Oratorio*
⊙ *Dunedin Consort/John Butt (Linn)*

Haydn – *Complete Symphonies*
⊙ *Heidelberg Symphony Orchestra/Thomas Fey (Hänssler Classics)*

World-weariness

Sometimes we all wish that we were blissfully unaware of life's dangers, that we could live our lives in childlike, carefree wonder. The poet William Blake knew that was impossible – that with naivety came ignorance, vulnerability and associated dangers. Music, however, can hand us the key to a world of innocent bliss, free from corruption and ennui.

Part of that is down to music's keys. Much like herbs and spices in food, keys, or key signatures, can bring different flavours to music. Composers are able to choose from an array of 24 keys – 12 major and 12 minor – to give their music a particular character. They might choose D major, for instance, for its optimism, A flat major for its sumptuousness tempered with a slight unease, or G minor for a touch of tragedy. For naivety, they will generally head to C major, the key denuded of sharps and flats, the purest, most childlike key of all – perfect for music of innocent expression. John Lennon's 'Imagine', for instance, a song that wears its naive idealism on its sleeve ('Imagine no possessions, I wonder if you can'), is written in C major.

Wolfgang Amadeus Mozart revels in the simplicity of one of the most famous children's songs of all, 'Twinkle, twinkle, little star' – or, in this case, its French setting, 'Ah! vous dirai-je, maman'. By scoring it in C major, Mozart signals his intentions to keep on a naive path, and despite its challenging passagework, it is playful, wide-eyed and free. Johann Sebastian Bach innately understood the connection between C major and innocence, too – the opening prelude of *The Well-Tempered Clavier* is one of his most technically accessible pieces, perfect for a child beginner and harmonically complex enough to maintain interest. As with the opening movement of his *Cello Suite No. 1*, Bach brilliantly combines simplicity and musical perfection.

W

Keys are just one way that composers achieve this light atmosphere. Scoring is another. At the end of Gustav Mahler's *Symphony No. 4* sits the song 'Das Himmlische Leben' ('This Heavenly Life'), a child's vision of heaven. Composed for soprano but intended to be performed with a bright, simple voice, the movement's description of heaven as a child's paradise is accompanied by jingling bells and a gorgeous, life-affirming theme. And at the start of Sergei Prokofiev's story for children, *Peter and the Wolf*, Peter ventures without a care in the world into the meadow behind his grandfather's house, accompanied by a richly scored melody for strings, its frolicking nature evoking both the beauty of spring and the innocence of youth.

RECOMMENDED LISTENING

Mozart – 12 Variations on 'Ah! vous dirai-je, maman'
⊙ *Kristian Bezuidenhout (piano) (Harmonia Mundi)*

Bach – 'Prelude No. 1' from Book I of *The Well-Tempered Clavier*
⊙ *Till Fellner (piano) (ECM)*

Mahler – *Symphony No. 4*
⊙ *Budapest Festival Orchestra/Iván Fischer (Channel Classics)*

Prokofiev – *Peter and the Wolf*
⊙ *David Bowie (narrator), Philadelphia Orchestra/Eugene Ormandy (Sony)*

W

Worry

Francis Poulenc's music veers wildly between clownish frivolousness and deep religious conviction, a contradiction that earned him the label 'half monk, half rascal'. On the one hand, the French composer was highly influenced by the irreverent music of Erik Satie (see page 81) and the neo-classical brashness of Igor Stravinsky (see page 106). Together, these heady influences, coupled with Poulenc's sense of mischief, resulted in works as ebullient and irrepressible as the ballet *Les Biches*, or the *Organ Concerto*, with its fairground frolics that cock a snook at Bach. The final movement of the *Trio for Oboe, Bassoon and Piano* is hilarious from start to finish.

On the other hand, Poulenc was a deeply sensitive man whose disastrous love life and grief at the premature death of his friend and fellow composer Pierre-Octave Ferroud produced works of searing religious and emotional depth. Listen to the *Litanies à la Vierge Noire* for female choir and organ, or the *Stabat Mater* for Poulenc at his most anguished – a composer with a gift for writing music of exquisite beauty.

Lurking between the introspection and hijinks is music of delightful insouciance – breezy, cheery, carefree works that seem to celebrate the joys of youth. The place to find these oases is mostly Poulenc's solo piano music, much of which is imbued with a Mozartian artlessness. Take the first of the *Trois novelettes* from 1927. Written in C major, its childlike innocence is apparent from the opening note, its relaxed, friendly mood ruffled just once or twice by brief hints of playfulness. For Poulenc at his happiest and most worry-free, listen to the *Soirées de Nazelles*, written between 1930 and 1936 – miniature improvisations played while the composer gazed fondly at portraits of his close friends. The overriding feelings of contented good humour in both works, music

W

that glances both forward and back, are a constant source of pleasure. Their nonchalance is entirely infectious.

RECOMMENDED LISTENING

Poulenc – *Soirées de Nazelles*

⊙ *Pascal Rogé (piano) (Decca)*

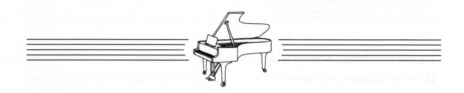

Y

Youthfulness (yearning for)

Do you sometimes wonder what it would be like to regain your youth? Without the school exams, of course, or the acne, or the angst surrounding boyfriends or girlfriends, or the peer pressures or the social awkwardness. Yes, it would be terrible.

But don those rose-tinted specs once again and imagine a world where youth equals freedom, beauty, naivety, uninterrupted playtime, promise and all those things we yearn for now that childhood has sailed. To help us in our impossible dreams, there are pieces of music we can turn to in which composers have captured perfectly the essence of youth, whether homages to childhood, reminders of student days, evocations of halcyon summers, or pieces that simply evoke the spirit of youth through their exquisite artlessness. Here are five pieces to remind you of the more idyllic moments in your past.

Schumann – *Kinderszenen ('Scenes from Childhood')*
Although the titles for each of the collection's 13 pieces were added afterwards, Robert Schumann beautifully captures the dreams, fears, playfulness and vulnerabilities of childhood. Schumann's wife, Clara, noted that he often seemed 'like a child' himself.

⊙ *Marc-André Hamelin (piano) (Hyperion)*

Debussy – *Children's Corner*

Although originally scored for solo piano, André Caplet's orchestration of *Children's Corner* is a frothy, spirited delight with its delicate portrait of a porcelain doll, 'Serenade for the doll', and a lullaby of an elephant who lived at a Paris zoo during Debussy's childhood (see also page 64).

⊙ *Jean-Efflam Bavouzet (piano) (Chandos)*

Brahms – *Academic Festival Overture*

Written as a thank you for the honorary PhD he received from the University of Breslau in 1879, Johannes Brahms's short orchestral work incorporates German student drinking songs, including 'Gaudeamus Igitur' ('Let's Celebrate').

⊙ *Gewandhaus Orchestra/Herbert Blomstedt (Pentatone)*

Elgar – *The Wand of Youth*

The tunes in Edward Elgar's beautifully orchestrated suites were originally written for a play put on by young members of his family. They combine cartoonish fun and charming sentiment with touches of mischief, and they draw on the composer's own tendency to yearn for the past.

⊙ *Hallé/Mark Elder (Hallé)*

Britten – *Simple Symphony*

'Boisterous Bourrée', 'Playful Pizzicato', 'Sentimental Sarabande' and 'Frolicsome Finale' are the movements that make up Benjamin Britten's sparkling orchestral work, based on music he wrote between the ages of nine and twelve. Impressions of youth straight from the horse's mouth.

⊙ *English Chamber Orchestra/Benjamin Britten (Decca)*

Y

Z

Zen (deficiency in)

Originating in 6th-century China, Zen is a Buddhist philosophy that encourages a return to our original nature through meditation and activities (painting, gardening, music, calligraphy and many more) that can promote inner peace and enhance concentration. Today, however, Zen has become a catch-all word for calmness and self-awareness, both of which we can all agree are in short supply. Of course, there are many other ancient arts and philosophies that also focus on physical, mental and spiritual well-being, and classical musicians have embraced many of them as ways to relax, to keep their bodies in good shape and to prepare themselves mentally for gruelling performances ahead.

King of meditation was the yoga-practising violinist Yehudi Menuhin, who once conducted the Berlin Philharmonic with his feet while standing on his head. Swiss pianist Andreas Haefliger has used the ancient Chinese martial art of Shaolin kung fu to help him develop core strength to achieve the subtlest of piano touches, while conductor Hugo Ticciati indulges daily in a series of physical and breathing exercises after taking a cold shower, all of which he credits with adding spontaneity and risk-taking to his playing and to his life in general.

Composers throughout the centuries have explored Eastern philosophies, often incorporating their texts and music into their own works. Richard Wagner was fascinated by Buddhism, for instance, and even sketched out (but never completed) an opera based on legends found in Eugène Burnouf's 1844 book, *Introduction to the History of Buddhism*. Gustav Holst's interest in the *Rig Veda*, an ancient collection of over 1,000 Hindu Sanskrit hymns, inspired him to compose, among other works, the beautiful, four-part *Choral Hymns from the Rig Veda*, scored for various combinations of voices and instruments. The long list of later 20th-century composers influenced by Zen Buddhism includes Philip Glass, Steve Reich, John Tavener, John Cage, Per Nørgård, Lou Harrison and Jonathan Harvey, whose *...towards a pure land* describes 'a state of mind beyond suffering, where there is no grasping' and 'a model of the world to which we can aspire'. It is a beautiful work in which to lose yourself – hypnotic, almost formless – and perfect for regaining your own state of Zen.

RECOMMENDED LISTENING

Harvey – *...towards a pure land*
⊙ *BBC Scottish Symphony Orchestra/Ilan Volkov (NMC)*

Notes

'disrupted families, severed...'
(**Bewilderment**, p.26): David Metzer,
'The New York Reception of "Pierrot
lunaire": The 1923 Premiere and Its
Aftermath', *The Musical Quarterly,* vol.78, no.4
(Winter 1994), p.669.

'the sound equivalent...', 'soup of vapid...',
'it renders me still...', 'trickery without the
magic...', 'we wait...' (**Boredom**, p.28):
'Boring pieces', *BBC Music Magazine*, August
2011, p.38.

'Many, many times...' (**Boredom**, p.28):
Lorena A Hickok, 'Rachmaninoff Admits
Composing Prelude, But He's Sorry He Did
It', *Minneapolis Tribune*, 11 November 1921.

'I feel I am the most unhappy...' (**Despair**,
p.37): Deborah Hayden, *Pox: Genius, Madness
and the Mysteries of Syphilis* (New York: Basic
Books, 2004), p.114.

'When I woke up...' (**Devotion, lack of**,
p.41): Martin Gregor-Dellin and Dietrich
Mack, ed., *Cosima Wagner's Diaries, Volume 1:
1869–1877*, trans. Geoffrey Skelton (New
York: Harcourt Brace Jovanovich, 1976),
p.312.

'What I shit is better...' (**Disappointment**,
p.43): Alex Ross, 'Deus ex musica', *The
New Yorker*, 13 October 2014, https://www.
newyorker.com/magazine/2014/10/20/deus-
ex-musica, accessed 18 June 2021.

'Of course, I could scribble...' (**Disdain**,
p.45): Jan Swafford, *Mozart: The Reign of Love*
(London: Faber & Faber, 2020), p.228.

'The Concerto I'll write him...' (**Disdain**,
p.45): Swafford, *Mozart*, p.229.

'In December 1927...' (**Embarrassment**,
p.47): Alexandra Coghlan, *Carols From King's*
(London: Random House, 2016), pp.156–7.

'which is generally accepted...' (**Exhaustion**,
p.49): A Szabo, A Small, and M Leigh, 'The
effects of slow-and fast-rhythm classical
music on progressive cycling to voluntary
physical exhaustion', *The Journal of Sports
Medicine and Physical Fitness*, vol. 39, no.3
(1999), p.220–25.

'the most amiable, harmless anger...'
(**Grumpiness**, p.68): Quoted in Konrad
Wolf, ed., *On Music and Musicians*, trans.
Paul Rosenfeld (Berkeley, CA: University
of California Press, 1946), p.105.

'would have been a great composer...'
(**Grumpiness**, p.68): Laura Ward, *Put
Downs: A Collection of Acid Wit* (London:
Robson Books, 2004), p.105.

'the best, and, in particular...' (**Heartbreak,
wallowing in**, p.73): Timothy L Jackson,
Tchaikovsky: Symphony No. 6 (Pathétique)
(Cambridge: Cambridge University Press,
1999), p.1.

'I have allowed my heart...' (**Inadequacy**,

p.87): Jerrold Northrop Moore, *Edward Elgar: A Creative Life* (Oxford: Oxford University Press, 1984), p.334.

'The impression made on my heart..' (**Infatuation**, p.88): Peter Raby, *Fair Ophelia: A Life of Harriet Smithson Berlioz* (Cambridge: Cambridge University Press, 1982), p.76.

'which should be of such...' (**Insomnia**, p.91): Martin Geck, *Johann Sebastian Bach: Life and Work* (Orlando, FL: Harcourt, 2006), p.229.

'beset by boredom...' (**Isolation**, p.93): Walter Winzenburger, 'Translation from Gerber's Historischbiographisches Lexikon der Tonkünstler (1790)', *Bach*, vol.1, no.2 (April 1970), p.29.

'Truly there would be a reason...' (**Mental Breakdown, understanding**, p.106): John Warrack, *Tchaikovsky* (London: Hamilton, 1973), p.125.

'I have once more begun...' (**Moodiness**, p.110): Felix Mendelssohn, letter to Fanny Mendelssohn, February 1831, quoted in *Letters of Felix Mendelssohn Bartholdy*, trans. Grace Jane Wallace (Boston: Oliver Ditson and Co., 1929), p.115.

'Never compose anything unless...' (**Passion**, p.121): Imogen Holst, *The Music of Gustav Holst* (London: Oxford University Press, 1968), p.73.

'I'm not starving...' (**Passion**, p.121): Mosco Carner, *Puccini: A Critical Biography* (New York: Alfred A Knopf, 1959), p.26.

'endless repetition...': (**Procrastination**, p.127): Matthew Boyden, *The Rough Guide to Opera* (London: Rough Guides, 2007), p.167.

'a row of braided...' (**Rebelliousness**, p.132): Thomas Forrest Kelly, *First Nights: Five Musical Premieres* (London: Yale University Press, 2000), p.290.

'Is he too, then...' (**Regret**, p.133): John Suchet, *Beethoven: The Man Revealed* (New York: Atlantic Monthly Press, 2012), p.149.

'slipt many opportunities...' (**Sadness**, p.139): Henry Peacham, *The Compleat Gentleman* (London: F. Constable, 1622).

'bankers and tradesmen...', 'the most triumphant laughter...' (**Schadenfreude**, p.141): Ernst Krause, *Richard Strauss: The Man and His Work* (Boston: Crescendo Publishing Company, 1969), pp.236, 237.

'He used to visit hospitals...' (**Selfishness**, p.143): Ronald Taylor, *Franz Liszt: The Man and the Musician* (London: Grafton Books, 1986), p.32.

'no one among contemporary artists...' (**Selfishness**, p.144): Taylor, *Franz Liszt*, pp.220–21.

'If you're ever walking...' (**Weepiness**, p.173): Christopher Grogan, *Edward Elgar: Music, Life and Landscapes* (Barnsley: Pen & Sword), p.205.

Index

Acknowledgements

There are so many emotions involved in writing a book. Elation at getting the project off the ground, then the inevitable daily procrastination and a constant blend of frustration, anxiety, stress, laziness and determination. Finally, joy and relief when deadlines are met and a draft makes its way to the publisher. In many ways, you could say that *Symphonies for the Soul* carried itself along its own journey, and, although music played its inevitable part, I have a few people to thank for helping me cross the finish line. Firstly, my parents David and Susan for first sparking and nurturing my musical passions, and my elder brother Charlie for initially setting the bar so high. Thanks, too, to my parents-in-law, Mike and Annie, for their generosity and patience, and to Daniel Jaffé for his inspiring replies to my cryptic emails. I couldn't, however, have written this book without the encouragement, constructive criticism and love of my darling wife, Caroline, to whom, along with our two dear children, I dedicate this book.

About the Author

Oliver Condy is a musician, editor and music journalist with 20 years of experience in music publishing. Until 2021, he was the editor of *BBC Music Magazine*, the world's best-selling classical music magazine where, during 17 years at the helm, he oversaw more than 220 issues. He is a regular contributor to BBC Radio 3's Saturday morning programme *Record Review*. Oliver is an organist, performing recitals from time to time.